Sex in China

Studies in Sexology in Chinese Culture

PERSPECTIVES IN SEXUALITY
Behavior, Research, and Therapy

Series Editor: RICHARD GREEN
University of California at Los Angeles

Sex in China

Studies in Sexology in Chinese Culture

Fang Fu Ruan

The Institute for Advanced Study of Human Sexuality
San Francisco, California

With the editorial collaboration of
Molleen Matsumura

Alin Foundation Institute
Berkeley, California

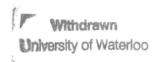
PLENUM PRESS • NEW YORK AND LONDON

Library of Congress Cataloging-in-Publication Data

Ruan, Fang-fu.
    Sex in China : studies in sexology in Chinese culture / Fang Fu
Ruan with the collaboration of Molleen Matsumura.
        p.   cm. -- (Perspectives in sexuality)
    Includes bibliographical references and index.
  • ISBN 0-306-43860-7
    1. Sexology--China.   I. Matsumura, Molleen.   II. Title.
III. Series.
HQ60.J83 1991
306'.0951--dc20   91-23139
                                                                        CIP

ISBN 0-306-43860-7

Printed in the United States of America

Series Editor's Comment

Less than a year before the 1989 massacre in Tiananmen Square, I lectured on human sexuality at Peking Union Medical College. I described my research on the nonsexual behaviors of young boys that predicted later homosexuality. I asked the physicians in the audience whether comparable childhood behaviors were found among Chinese boys. I was told that there are no homosexuals in China. How exceptional, if true. Clearly, there was a need for a candid account of sex in China.

I invited Professor Ruan to write this book when we first met. The scope of his scholarship and personal experience is exceptional.

China is a nation with a meticulously recorded sexual past, a culture where ancient values confront contemporary politics.

China is a nation of erotic paradox:

Centuries ago, sexuality was glorified—it was life enhancing, even granting immortality. Today's political climate is one of sexual repression.

Vivid portrayals of the sexual paraphilias were recorded hundreds of years ago. Today, China shuts down 42 publishers of erotic materials and seizes over 100,000 "pornographic" books in a single city. In a nation that celebrated erotic art, the death penalty awaits modern "traffickers in pornography."

This is a country where social dancing is restricted, but 80 percent of the people approve of premarital sex. A wedding night instructional manual has a first printing of four million copies.

For sexologists, China teaches the history of human sexuality over two millennia. Here is the full range of sexual expression, embedded in the contexts of changing politics and ancient and modern religion.

A quarter of the world lives here.

With Professor Ruan's work, Westerners need no longer have a blind spot in their view of Eastern sexuality.

RICHARD GREEN

Foreword

China today is sexually (and in many other ways) a very repressive society, yet ancient China was very different. Some of the earliest surviving literature of China is devoted to discussions of sexual topics, and the sexual implications of the Yin and Yang theories common in ancient China continue to influence Tantric and esoteric sexual practices today far distant from their Chinese origins.

In recent years, a number of books have been written exploring the history of sexual practices and ideas in China, but most have ended the discussion with ancient China and have not continued up to the present time. Fang Fu Ruan first surveys the ancient assumptions and beliefs, then carries the story to present-day China with brief descriptions of homosexuality, lesbianism, transvestism, transsexualism, and prostitution, and ends with a chapter on changing attitudes toward sex in China today.

Dr. Ruan is well qualified to give such an overview. Until he left China in the 1980s, he was a leader in attempting to change the repressive attitudes of the government toward human sexuality. He wrote a bestselling book on sex in China, and had written to and corresponded with a number of people in China who considered him as confidant and advisor about their sex problems. A physician and medical historian, Dr. Ruan's doctoral dissertation was a study of the history of sex in China.

What appears most evident is just how complicated a topic sex can be. Though sex is a biological function, the expression of sexuality is influenced by psychological, sociological, cultural, and historical factors. Chinese attitudes toward sex have never been quite the same as Western ones. It is also evident that repression of and hostility to sex—as has existed at various times in China, most recently under the Maoist government—can drive discussion of sex underground, but even underground there remains a great hunger for information about sex. Though such repression and its sequelae in lack of public discussion makes information about sex practices more difficult for the historian to ferret out, it seems clear that repression never eliminated homosexuality, prostitution, transvestism, or any other of the expressions of sexuality known to Western sexologists. Perhaps when China again becomes somewhat more open in the discussion of sexuality, the Chinese will be able to turn to Dr. Ruan's book for information about sexuality, not only in their ancient past, but also in the period of the 1970s and 1980s, where his knowledge is based on his own personal investigations.

In sum, *Sex in China* is a welcome contribution to the sexological literature.

VERN L. BULLOUGH

Amherst, New York

Preface

Though more than ten years have passed since China officially opened its doors to the Western world, this giant nation, with its population numbering in the billions, remains a land of mystery. Perhaps the deepest mysteries are those concerning sexual emotions and practices—forbidden territory to the Chinese themselves.

For the first 4,000 years of Chinese history, the prevailing Yin-Yang philosophy was the basis of open and positive attitudes toward human sexuality and a correspondingly rich sexological and erotic literature. However, the most recent 1,000 years of China's history have been characterized by repression and censorship which make the researcher's task extremely difficult. "Respectable" scholars dared not address the topic of sex; all materials relating to sex, including ancient medical classics, vibrant fiction, and wonderful paintings, were censored and destroyed. Even the religiously motivated sexual treatises of the Taoists were almost completely lost. The situation in contemporary China is even worse. With the exception of a few government publications, materials concerning sexuality are strictly forbidden; in the worst case, an individual convicted of production of "pornography" may be sentenced to death.

Sex in China is an attempt to overcome these obstacles in order to provide the reader with a survey of sexual life in China from 3,000 years ago to the present. A strictly chronological presentation is unnecessarily restrictive. Instead, I have traced the history of a number of areas of sexological interest, including sexual philosophy, classical sexological literature, Taoist sexual myths and techniques, erotic fiction, prostitution, male and female homosexuality, transvestism, transsexualism, and political regulation of sexuality and sexual rights. In treating each of these topics, it has been my concern to outline the great contributions of the Chinese people to sexology and sexual literature, to elucidate the processes by which an open, sex-positive culture became negative and repressive, and to demonstrate the ineffectiveness of repressive governmental policies, whether practiced by imperial regimes or the current dictatorship.

The thoughtful reader will wonder how it is possible to develop an accurate portrait of a nation whose government, consistent with a general denigration of sexuality, fails to provide nationwide statistics on sexual matters. Some of this information has been inferred from statistics developed by national and local governmental agencies concerning related topics such as the incidence of sexually transmitted diseases and marital statistics. Such data are reported in a variety of publications both in China and abroad, and, while it is difficult to evaluate their accuracy, they can be compared for consistency. In light of my personal experiences as a physician and sexologist, it is clear that the information permits conclusions about major social trends.

I left China for the United States at the end of 1985. If I had remained, I could never have written a book such as this. I am deeply grateful to my friends in China and to my American and Chinese friends in states as diverse as Texas, Utah, New York, Indiana, and California, who helped me come here to live and work.

I am especially grateful to Professors Vern L. Bullough and Bonnie Bullough, who invited me to stay in their home for six months in 1988; their rich library, their time, their understanding, and their hospitality and friendship have been invaluable for my study and writing. I am grateful, too, to Professor Robert Theodore McIlvenna, who generously permitted me to study and work at the Institute for Advanced Study of Human Sexuality in San Francisco, California.

I would like to express my thanks to Professor Richard Green, who invited me to write this book, and Eliot Werner and Herman Makler of Plenum Press, who oversaw its prompt publication. Dr. Kenneth Matsumura gave his encouragement and insightful comments on the manuscript. Mrs. Molleen Matsumura skillfully collaborated with me in editing the manuscript for publication; her assistance was invaluable in rendering masses of arcane data into readable prose and in helping maintain the desired balance between advocacy and objectivity. They all have my heartfelt thanks for introducing me to the world of English-language scholarship.

FANG FU RUAN

San Francisco, California

Contents

Chapter 4

Sexual Techniques of the Taoists: Myths and Methods 49

Chapter 5

Prostitution in Chinese Society: From Acceptance to
Persecution 69

Chapter 6

Classical Chinese Erotica: Then and Now 85

Chapter 1

Introduction

For centuries, the Chinese people thought of their country as the center of the world; indeed, "China," in the Chinese language, is "zhong guo," which literally means "Central Kingdom." This phrase has a certain ring of truth when one considers that China has an enormous land area, the world's largest population, and the longest recorded history of any nation.

China's civilization is remarkable not only for its age but also for its continuity, in which the written language has been an important factor. The written language consists of thousands of written characters or "ideograms," each of which represents a single idea. Combinations of ideograms also represent specific ideas; for example, combining the ideogram "nu," meaning "woman, girl, daughter, or female," with the ideogram "zi," meaning "man, boy, son, or male," creates the ideogram "hao," meaning "good, nice." (The combined ideogram indicates that one who has both a son and a daughter is good, and that to unite or combine an individual man and woman, or male and female essences, is desirable.) Thus speakers of varying local dialects are able to communicate in writing. Since it has changed very little in the last 2,000 years, the written language has functioned as a unifying force across time as well as space. Among other aspects of Chinese civilization, the use of ideograms spread to Korea and Japan, and many literary classics which can no longer be obtained in China have been identified in Japanese and Korean collections.

CHINA'S OLDEST SEX LITERATURE

The world's oldest sex handbooks are Chinese. We do not know when the Chinese began recording their sexual knowledge and practices, but the oldest extant texts date from about 200 B.C. (The books next described will be discussed in detail in Chapter 3.)

The oldest texts were discovered in 1973 at the Ma-wang-tui Han Tomb No. 3, Ma-wang-tui, Chang-sa, Hunan province. The date of the burial in this tomb was 168 B.C. The interment included fourteen medical texts, three of them sexological works: *Ten Questions and Answers* (Shiwan), *Methods of Intercourse between Yin and Yang* (He-yin-yang-fang), and *Lectures on the Super Tao in the Universe* (Tian-xia-zhi-tao-tan). (Some of these texts will be discussed in Chapter 3.)

In different periods from before the Han dynasty until the end of the Tang dynasty, more than twenty sex handbooks were produced and circulated. Those still extant are listed in Table 1–1. The importance of these texts and other Chinese sexual materials is best understood in the context of Chinese history, which is briefly outlined here.

SKETCH OF CHINESE HISTORY

Our knowledge of China's earliest history is a blend of archeology and mythology. The most interesting of the remote predecessors of the Chinese is "Peking man," a forerunner of modern humans. Fossils of this species were discovered in 1927 in a cave at Zhoukoudian (Chou Kou Tien) about thirty miles southwest of the Chinese capital Beijing (Peking) (Reischauer and Fairbank, 1960). According to the latest measurement made in 1989, Peking man lived approximately 578,000 years ago. (*People's Daily*, Overseas Edition, October 23, 1989). The species name has been variously latinized as *Sinanthropus pekinensis*, *Pithecanthropus pekinensis*, and *Homo erectus pekinensis*. Whatever the appellation, it possessed hominid fea-

Table 1–1. Ancient Chinese Sex Handbooks Still Extant

English title	Chinese title	Date of origin[a]
Canon of the Immaculate Girl	Su Nu Ching	Han dynasty
Prescriptions of the Immaculate Girl	Su Nu Fang	Han dynasty
Important Matters of the Jade Chamber	Yu Fang Chih Yao	Pre-Sui dynasty (before A.D. 581— possibly during the fourth century)
Secret Instructions Concerning the Jade Chamber	Yu Fang Pi Chueh	Same
Book of the Mystery-Penetrating Master	Tung Hsuan Tzu	Pre-Tang dynasty (before A.D. 618, possibly the fifth century)
Poetical Essay on the Supreme Joy	Ta Lo Fu	A.D. ninth Century[b]

[a]Dates of dynasties are listed in Table 1–2.
[b]This is the only text whose author is known. The author, Pai Hsing-Chien, lived from A.D. 775–826.

tures: erect posture, considerable cranial capacity (average 1,075 cc), and the capability of making and using tools and implements (K. C. Chang, 1977). Fossils of this species have also been found in Java and Africa. They were occasional cave dwellers who made stone tools and used fire.

China's popular history reaches back into the mists of legend. Mythical kings are said to have invented fire, architecture, clothing, cooking, medical arts, marriage, and methods of government.

Chinese mythology began with Pan Ku, the creator, who was followed by a succession of four culture heroes credited with having taught the Chinese people the arts of civilization. According to legend, You Cao Shi taught people to build wooden houses; Sui Ren Shi taught the use of the fire drill; Fu Xi Shi taught hunting, fishing with nets, and cattle-raising; and Shen Nong Shi taught herbal medicine and techniques of cultivating grain. These culture heroes were followed by the legendary "Wu Ti" (Five Emperors), including the Yellow Emperor (Huang Ti), Emperor Yao, and Emperor Xun. The Yellow Emperor is mentioned frequently in traditional Chinese medical and sexological books.

The reign of the mythical Five Emperors was always described as preceding the Xia dynasty, the first dynasty of which we have historical records; the founding of the Xia dynasty was long thought to mark the beginning of Chinese history. Recently, however, Chinese archeologists working in western Liaoning province between 1979 and 1986 discovered the first reliable archeological evidence of Chinese culture before the Xia dynasty. Their discoveries included a goddess temple and sacrificial altar built over 5,000 years ago. The culture of this period is now known as the "Hongshan (Red Mountain)." Nonetheless, the Xia still holds the title of "First Dynasty."

Like his mythical predecessors, the first Xia emperor, Emperor Yu, was considered a model emperor of exceptional wisdom and virtue. Yu, by leaving his throne to his son, originated the system of succession in which an emperor was succeeded by a member of his own family, usually a son.

The second dynasty, dating from the sixteenth to eleventh centuries B.C., was the Shang, or Yin. The discovery of thousands of inscribed bones and tortoise shells in An-yang, Hunan province between 1928 and 1937 has enabled historians to date the Shang dynasty with reasonable certainty.

The third dynasty, the Zhou, was subdivided into the Western Zhou (1111–771 B.C.) and Eastern Zhou (770–221 B.C.). Eastern Zhou was further subdivided into the Spring-and-Autumn period (770–476 B.C.) and the Warring States period (475–221 B.C.). Beginning in the Zhou dynasty, China already had written historical records and books. This rich and significant era of Chinese history witnessed the birth of the "zhuzi baijia" (literally, "one hundred various schools"), the major Chinese philosophical schools, including Confucianism, Taoism, and Legalism, as well as the earliest codifications of medicine and sexology.

Confucius (551–479 B.C.) codified previous philosophical theories, and two hundred years later Mencius expounded and championed Confucius' ideas. Together they laid the theoretical foundations of Confucian philosophy, whose core conception is an ethical vision of orderly social relations. Confucius himself expressed a rather positive view of human sexuality, as will be discussed in Chapter 2, and it was not until much later that sexual conservatism became a feature of Neo-Confucian philosophy.

Yin-Yang is another major philosophical concept developed during the Zhou dynasty. It was Tsou Yen (305–240 B.C.) who founded the "Yin-Yang School," though the concepts of Yin and Yang had been discussed by various philosophers long before his time. The concepts of Yin and Yang may be found in the majority of important Chinese classics, including such major classics of Confucianism as the *I-Ching* and such Taoist classics as the *Tao-te-ching*. Thus, Yin-Yang philosophy is among the most important unifying concepts of Chinese culture. The Yin-Yang concept is so integral to Chinese culture that any cultural study, especially a sexological study, must include an explanation of it. The essentials of Yin-Yang philosophy and its relevance to sexological studies are explained in Chapters 2, 3, and 4.

During the two dynasties following the Zhou dynasty—the Chin (255–206 B.C.) and Han (206 B.C.–A.D. 220) dynasties—the boundaries of the Chinese nation were extended to the south to include the modern provinces of Fujian, Guangdong, and Yunnan, and the present nation of Vietnam. Bounded on the east by the China Sea, on the north by the desert of Mongolia, and on the west by the Pamir Plateau, China had become a great nation. The predominant people were Han, sharing common origins, appearance, written and spoken language, and customs. During subsequent invasions, the conquerors found that they could not dominate the Han and were eventually assimilated by them.

By the time of the Han dynasty, the Chinese culture, medicine, and sexology were already well developed. Table 1–2 (adapted from Day, 1978) summarizes the major actors and events of subsequent dynasties.

Some historians divide Chinese history into three periods: the Formative Age (Prehistory–206 B.C.), the Early Empire (206 B.C.–A.D. 960), and the Later Empire (960–1850) (Hucher, 1975). This division is useful in the study of the history of Chinese sexuality and sexology. Broadly speaking, Chinese attitudes toward human sexuality were open and positive during the Formative and Early Empire ages, but increasingly closed and negative during the Later Empire period. During the ensuing years from 1850 to the present, which might be termed the Modern Period, negative sex attitudes and policies continued under three radically dif-

Table 1–2. Chinese History and Culture in Brief

Dynasties	Approximate dates	Significant figures and events
Legendary Period	2852–2197 B.C.	
Primitive Dynasties	2197–221 B.C.	
Xia [Hsia]	1994–1523 B.C.	Bronze casting
Shang (Yin)	1523–1027 B.C.	Oracle Bones of Yin
Zhou [Chou]	1027–221 B.C.	Lao Tzu, Confucius, Mencius
Ancient Dynasties	221 B.C.–A.D. 618	
Qin (Chin)		Building of Great Wall
Han	207 B.C.–A.D. 220	Confucianism established; Buddhism introduced
Three Kingdoms	220–265	
Jin [Chin]	265–420	
North & South	420–589	Buddhism well developed
Sui	589–618	
Medieval Dynasties	A.D. 618–1368	
Tang [T'ang][a]	618–905	Buddhism flourishing; arts and literature develop; printing invented
Five Dynasties	905–960	
Song [Sung]	960–1279	Neo-Confucian philosophy
Yuan [Mongol]	1280–1368	Marco Polo visits China
Modern Dynasties	A.D. 1368–1911	
Ming	1368–1644	Painting, industry, all arts flourish
Ching [Manchu]	1644–1911	T'aiping Rebellion; Opium War

[a]An apostrophe within a word ("T'ang" vs. "Tang," for example) is sometimes used to indicate the pronunciation in spoken Chinese. Most of these have been eliminated from the text for convenience. Also, the spellings used in the text are generally those most familiar to Americans—for example, "Sung" dynasty rather than "Song" dynasty.

ferent regimes: the late Ching dynasty, the Republic of China, and the People's Republic of China. The nature and meaning of these differences will be discussed in depth in the following pages.

STUDIES OF CHINESE SEXOLOGY IN ENGLISH

R. H. van Gulik's *Sexual Life in Ancient China*

The first Westerner to succeed in producing an important study of Chinese sexuality was R. H. van Gulik. In 1951 he published a rare collection of Chinese erotic literature (see the following), and a decade later, he published his famous *Sexual Life in Ancient China* (1961), which is still the only standard, systematic, academic book concerning sexual life in ancient China. This was an enlarged and revised edition of his earlier, unusual *Erotic Colour Prints of the Ming Period, with an Essay on Chinese Sex Life from the Han to the Ch'ing Dynasty, B.C. 206–A.D. 1644* (Volume I: English text; Volume II: Chinese text; Volume III: reprint of the Hua-ying-chin-chen album) (private edition, Tokyo, Japan, 1951, limited to 50 copies).

Van Gulik tells an interesting story about the circumstances that led him to become a scholar of Chinese sexuality:

> In 1949 when I was serving as Counsellor of the Netherlands Embassy in Tokyo, I happened to find in a curio-shop a set of old Chinese printing blocks of a Ming erotic album, entitled Hua-ying-chin-chen ("Variegated Battle Arrays of the Flowery Camp)....
>
> Since such albums are now exceedingly rare, and important from both the artistic and the sociological point of view, I thought it my duty to make this material available to other research workers. My original plan was to have a few copies struck off from those blocks and publish them in a limited edition, adding a brief preface on the historical background of Chinese erotic art.

As van Gulik pursued his research, his "preface" grew into an essay of more than 200 pages, and when in 1951 he finally published *Erotic Colour Prints of the Ming Period, with an Essay on Chinese Sex Life from the Han to the Ch'ing Dynasty, B.C. 206–A.D. 1644*, it comprised three volumes. Since it contained reproductions of erotic prints and other material that van Gulik felt was most appropriate for a specialized audience, he limited the edition to fifty copies, all of which were presented to various Oriental and Western research institutions.

In 1956, at his publisher's request that he write a book on ancient Chinese sex and society, he decided to expand the historical commentary in his earlier book, modestly remarking of his pioneering work, "The present book is a mere outline,... this is the first book on the subject" (van Gulik, 1961).

The expanded text is enriched by material from a great number of primary sources and a bibliography locating the sexological references in a number of works devoted to other topics. Van Gulik included excerpts from many texts which are difficult to obtain, and his work benefits from insights gained during his years of residence in China.

J. Needham's *Science and Civilization in China*

Joseph Needham, a world-renowned scholar, biochemist, member of the Royal Academy, and a great British historian of Chinese science and technology, was another pioneering student of Chinese sexology. His *Science and Civilization in China* is a monumental work which will comprise seven volumes when completed (so far, five volumes have been published). Needham first discussed Taoist sexual technique as a special topic in the second volume (1956) and expanded his discussion considerably in the fifth volume (1983). The original study is especially noteworthy for its very good general description of Taoist sexual practices, which places them in their philosophical and historical context. Needham's bibliography, like van Gulik's, is an excellent resource guide. Needham's assertion that the Taoists accepted "the equality of women with men" has been modified by other researchers.

Other Works in English

From the 1950s to 1980s, several other books on Chinese sexuality and/or Chinese sexology were published, including Girchner (1957), Levy (1965, 1974), Ishihara and Levy (1968), Beurdeley *et al.* (1969), Etiemble (1970), Chou (1971), Humana and Jacobs (1971), J. Chang (1977, 1983), de Smedt (1981), Humana and Wu (1982), Chia (1984, 1986), and S. T. Chang (1986). In the same period, several books introduced classical Chinese erotic paintings, among them Kronhausen (1968, 1978), Rawsan (1968, 1981), Smith (1974), Franzblau and Etiemble (1977), and Douglas and Slinger (1981). Many of these books (see the references with annotations), though useful, are limited by either concentrating on a specialized topic or presenting a popular treatment of their subject. Some, by treating sexuality as a domain of pleasure independent of the changing contexts in medicine, religion, family life, reproductive strategies, or social control, effectively reinforce stereotypes of exotic Oriental cultures.

There were few bibliographies (Ishihara & Levy, 1968; Hallingby, 1981; Cheng, Furth, & Yip, 1984) which listed the English literature on Chinese sexuality. The items that were related to Chinese sexology and were included in them are very limited.

SIGNIFICANCE OF STUDIES OF CHINESE SEXUALITY

There is still much work to be done in the field of Chinese sexology. These studies are clearly relevant to a number of other fields, as next outlined.

Significance to Historians of Sexuality and Gender

For more than 2,000 years, the Chinese people have recorded information about the psychology and sociology of sex in a variety of genres. This information is not limited to specifically medical and sexological texts. For example, a wealth of information about gender roles is contained in two of the "Five Confucian Classics." One of these, *She King (The Book of Poetry)*, is the oldest repository of Chinese verse; it was probably compiled in the early sixth century B.C., and contains 305 poems and folk songs dating from the eleventh to the sixth centuries B.C.; the second, the *I-Ching (Book of Changes)*, is one of the oldest and most important philosophy books. Many novels and essays of the Tang, Sung, Ming, and Ching dynasties contained equally rich material about gender roles. Thus the study of China's sexological and erotic literature is indispensable to historical studies of sex, gender, and sex roles.

Significance to Sexology

A truly universal understanding of human sexuality must be based on a comparative sexology of many cultures. While the sexual beliefs and practices of many peoples are transmitted by oral traditions which may not be easily accessible to scholarship, the study of Oriental sexology is buttressed by a rich literature. The study of Chinese and Indian sexuality and sexology is the core academic field of Oriental sexology.

Oriental sexology has practical significance in addition to its historical value. Taoist sexual technique, for example, is of special interest. While some of these techniques appear frivolous in light of modern sexual knowledge, others remain valid and effective (for example, methods for delaying ejaculation).

Significance to Sinology

Sexual culture, especially when broadly construed to include the elaboration of gender roles, represents a major aspect of the entire social life of a country. Moreover, sexual relationships have influenced politics in both ancient and modern China. The study of sexual culture and the historical study of sex in China have been veiled in ignorance for centuries. A renewed study of these topics will inevitably enrich general sinology.

Significance to Sociology and Anthropology

Chinese culture has influenced neighboring cultures for millennia, and with the world's largest population, China will continue to play a major role in world culture. Thus the study of Chinese sexual practices will make a significant contribution to the sociology and anthropology of sex, gender, and sex roles.

Significance to Politics, Modernization, and Cultural Life in China

It is common knowledge that in today's mainland China, conservative and reformist factions are locked in a struggle for power. While these factions are bitter enemies in matters of politics and economics, they share a common attitude toward sexual matters. The two factions actually are, or at least pretend to be, equally conservative and ignorant in their approach to the question of sexual rights. The conservative faction continually accuses the reformers of being responsible for the introduction of prostitution, rape, and "sexual immorality." The reform wing defends itself by denouncing sexual freedom more loudly than the conservatives. The result is that the Chinese people suffer under a terribly repressive sex policy.

Any genuine political reform will have to include a changed sex policy. At the "Democracy Wall" in the winter of 1978–1979 and in nationwide demonstrations by university students in the winter of 1986–1987, some of China's bravest young people declared that a more open sex policy is crucial to the modernization of the country. The poem "Open Sex," translated in Chapter 9, typifies these young people's concerns.

This important topic has been closed to discussion for far too long, and if China's leaders cannot change their sexual attitudes, it will be impossible to achieve other vital social reforms. If reformist leaders will have the courage to point out that rates of prostitution and rape in China are comparable to those of other countries, they can effectively counter the conservative tactic of blaming these ills on progressive social reforms. They should also affirm that a more open sex policy might well decrease the incidence of prostitution and rape, as well as lead to improvements in other areas such as marital relations. Such a position would surely be welcomed by the Chinese people, strengthening resistance to conservative policies. Thus the systematic study of historical and modern Chinese sexuality can play an important role in bringing about social reforms and ridding the Chinese people of the burdens of sexual hypocrisy and inhumanity.

It is also very important that the historical, sociological, and biomedical study of Chinese sexuality will help to greatly improve the sexual life of the Chinese people. When serious academic studies demonstrate that in the most illustrious periods of Chinese history homosexuality was in high repute and a variety of heterosexual behaviors and erotic literature were quite common, the current government's claim that these are decadent Western imports will be effectively refuted. Thus precise and accurate knowledge can help strengthen the position of the common people in their struggle for basic sexual rights.

CONCLUSION: THE NEED FOR A MODERN SEXOLOGICAL STUDY

Although van Gulik's work (1961) remains the standard text on sexuality in Chinese history, it takes us only to the end of the Ming dynasty (A.D. 1644), and a number of important works dating from the periods he does cover were unavailable or undiscovered at the time he was writing. Sexological works written in about the last thousand years were prohibited by the reigning governments and have been very difficult to obtain.

All too many treatments of Chinese sexuality have been from a limited perspective, usually focusing on historical and literary approaches. Yet this is a broad and complex topic encompassing the fields of biology, medicine, psychology, sociology, anthropology, ethics, politics, and law, in addition to history and literature. It is time we saw more studies based on comprehensive sources, including newly discovered and rare materials, and analyzing their subject from all possible academic angles.

Chapter 2

The Harmony of Yin and Yang
Chinese Sexual Philosophy

THE YIN-YANG CONCEPT

The concept of Yin-Yang is essentially simple, yet its influence on Chinese culture has been extensive. There is no aspect of Chinese civilization—including philosophy, medicine, sexology, politics, government, literature, and art—that has not been touched by this simple, powerful idea. According to Yin-Yang philosophy, all objects and events are the products of two elements, forces, or principles: Yin, which is negative, passive, weak, and destructive, and Yang, which is positive, active, strong, and constructive. It is quite possible that the two sexes, whether conceived in terms of female and male essences, the different social roles of women and men, or the structural differences between female and male sex organs, are not only the most obvious results of the workings of Yin and Yang forces, but major sources from which the ancient Chinese derived these concepts as well. Certainly, it was very natural for the Yin-Yang doctrine to become the basis of Chinese sexual philosophy.

The Chinese have used the words Yin and Yang to refer to sexual organs and sexual behavior for several thousand years. Thus "Yin Fu" ("the door of Yin") means vulva, "Yin Dao" ("the passageway of Yin") means vagina, and "Yang Ju" ("the organ of Yang") means penis. The combination of these words into the phrases "Huo Yin Yang" or "Yin Yang Huo He," or "the union or combination of Yin and Yang," describes the act of sexual intercourse. These words were also used in constructing more abstract sexual terminology. According to Han Shu (*History of the*

Former Han) edited by Pan Ku (A.D. 32–92), the earliest terms referring to classical Chinese sexology were "Yin Dao" (or "Yin Tao"), meaning "the way of Yin," and "yang Yang fang," meaning "the method for maintaining Yang in good condition." (See Chapter 3.)

Because the Yin-Yang theory holds that the harmonious interaction of male and female principles is vital, it is the basis of an essentially open and positive attitude toward sexuality. The following passages from the classic *I-Ching*, which will be discussed in detail below, are representative of the traditional sex-positive viewpoint:

> The constant intermingling of Heaven and Earth gives shape to all things. The sexual union of man and woman gives life to all things.
> The interaction of one Yin and one Yang is called Tao (the Supreme Path or Order), the resulting constant generative process is called "change." (Translated by van Gulik, 1961)

These two passages are frequently quoted in later sex handbooks, where "one Yin" and "one Yang" always refer to a woman and a man. Thus, it was thought that any time a man and woman join in sexual intercourse, they are engaging in an activity that reflects and maintains the order of nature.

THE YIN-YANG CONCEPT IN TRADITIONAL CHINESE MEDICINE

Traditional Chinese medicine is based on the medical classic *Nei Jing*. This title, which is translated as "Internal Classic," or "Canon of Internal Medicine," is an abbreviation of the title *Huangdi Nei Jing*, or *The Yellow Emperor's Canon of Internal Medicine*. Although it is traditionally attributed to the legendary hero, it is known to be the work of various unknown authors who wrote during the Warring States Period (475–221 B.C.). It is the oldest and greatest medical classic extant in China, and its foundation is the Yin-Yang concept. Thus the anonymous author of Book 2 of *Nei Jing* asserts, "Yin-Yang is the way of heaven and earth, the boundaries of everything, the parents of change, the root and beginning of birth and destruction, the place of Gods. Treatment of disease should be based upon the root" (Book 2, Chapter 5: "Great Treatise on Yin-Yang Classifications of Natural Phenomena," translated by Lu, 1978).

The medical significance of the Yin and Yang principles differs somewhat from their significance in other areas of Chinese culture. In general, the Yin-Yang doctrine supported men's higher social status, since not only masculinity but also light, good fortune, and all that is desirable were associated with Yang, while darkness, evil, and femininity were associated with Yin. However, from the medical standpoint, both Yang and Yin were necessary and valuable—in fact, Yin might be considered even more important, being associated with the structural, or material, aspects of the human body.

In Chinese medicine, the patient's physical constitution, disease symptoms, and herbal and dietary remedies are all classified as Yin or Yang. For the purposes of this system, Yang is associated with exteriority, excess, and heat, and Yin is associated with interiority, deficiency, and cold. Illness is conceived as an imbalance of Yin and Yang elements, and all treatment is oriented to restoring a harmonious balance.

In diagnosis, for example, such symptoms as agitation, a dry tongue, deep breathing, and a full pulse are associated with Yang, and listlessness, a moist, swollen tongue, shallow breathing, and a weak pulse are associated with Yin. Even body odor and the appearance of the "moss" on the tongue are categorized as Yin or Yang. Foods are analyzed according to five flavors, five "energies," movements (outward or inward, downward or upward—for example, food that causes perspiration has "outward movement"), and actions. Thus cold or cool, rich, or moist foods are Yin, warm or hot, and dry are Yang. Sweetness, saltiness, sourness, bitterness, and other flavors are all classified. Of course, Yin and Yang characteristics may be combined in one food, and all must be considered together in determining whether a food is mildly or strongly Yin or Yang. (The same applies to disease symptoms.)

Once a person's constitution and symptoms are analyzed, it is possible to apply the advice given in Book 9 of *Nei Jing:*

> A cold disease should be heated up, a hot disease should be made cold, a warm disease should be cooled down, a cool disease should be warmed up, a dispersing disease should be constricted, an inhibiting disease should be dispersed, a dry disease should be lubricated, an acute disease should be slowed down, a hard disease should be softened, a crisp disease should be hardened, a weakening disease should be toned up, a strong disease should be sedated. (Translated by Lu, 1978)

These principles are applied in preventive care as well as treatment of disease. Thus, according to the Chinese way of thinking, a "balanced diet" is defined not in terms of proteins and carbohydrates, vitamins and minerals but of Yin and Yang qualities. Accordingly, a person with a hot physical constitution might be expected to drink tea, which has cold energy, while a person with a cold physical constitution would achieve balance by drinking coffee, which has a hot energy.

Once one understands the primacy of the medical principle of basing treatment and health maintenance on an effort to balance Yin and

Yang, the traditionally positive attitude toward sexual intercourse seems natural. Sexual intercourse, by giving the participants an opportunity to exchange and balance Yin and Yang energies, was sometimes even seen as a prerequisite to health.

THE *I-CHING*, YIN-YANG, AND SEX

The famous *I-Ching (Book of Changes)* is one of the earliest and most important Chinese classics, equally cherished in both the Confucian and the Taoist traditions. It is based on interpretation of prophetic symbols— the eight trigrams and sixty-four hexagrams. According to tradition, the eight trigrams were devised by the legendary ruler, Fu Xi Shi, and the sixty-four hexagrams by a historical figure, King Wen (1171–1122 B.C.); some other portions of the book are ascribed to King Wen or to Duke Zhou (d. 1094 B.C.) and to Confucius. Most scholars are skeptical of these attributions, but cannot agree as to when, and by whom, the book was written. Most likely it is the work of many authors, writing from as early as the sixth century B.C. to as late as the third century B.C. The book has a complex structure, consisting of the trigrams and hexagrams, basic interpretations accompanying these figures, commentaries on these interpretations, and layers of commentaries upon the commentaries.

The core texts consist of the sixty-four hexagrams and their interpretations. These hexagrams are based on the eight trigrams, each of which consists of three lines; each line is either divided or undivided, the divided representing Yin and the undivided representing Yang. Each of the eight trigrams corresponds to a set of natural phenomena—a direction, a natural element, a moral quality, and so forth. The eight trigrams are illustrated in Figure 2–1.

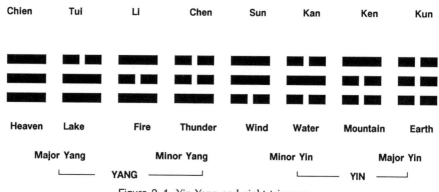

Figure 2–1. Yin-Yang and eight trigrams.

Each trigram is combined with another, one being placed above the other, to create the sixty-four hexagrams, which are supposed to symbolize all possible situations. For example, the sixty-fourth hexagram "Wei-Chi" (Incompletion), with the fire trigram over the water trigram, symbolizes that which is not yet completed or successfully accomplished.

The interpretations of the trigrams include abstract philosophical and ethical concepts which are the basis of much Chinese philosophical speculation. However, it is important to note that the *I-Ching* also contains explicit descriptions of sexual organs and sexual behaviors. In fact, the noted Chinese scholars Qian Xuian-tung and Guo Mo-ruo have pointed out that the basic elements of the hexagrams, the divided (Yin) and the undivided (Yang) lines, represent the vulva and penis, respectively (Guo, 1954; Qian, 1982; Jiang, 1988).

Thanks to its utilization of the Yin-Yang concept, the *I-Ching* is permeated by sexual imagery at both the abstract and concrete levels, in both Taoist and Confucian expressions. The earlier-quoted statement, "The constant intermingling of Heaven and Earth gives shape to all things. The sexual union of man and woman gives life to all things" (van Gulik, 1961) is given a typically Taoist expression in the comment, "The interaction of one Yin and one Yang is called Tao (the Supreme Path or Order); the resulting constant generative process is called 'change'." In another text (translated by Chan, 1963), essentially the same idea is attributed to Confucius: "Heaven is high, the earth is low, and thus Chien (Heaven) and Kun (Earth) are fixed.... The way of Chien constitutes the male, while the way of Kun constitutes the female. Chien knows the great beginning, and Kun acts to bring things to completion." Another comment attributed to Confucius encapsulates the concept that combining Yin and Yang creates a necessary and healthful balance: "Chien and Kun are indeed the gate of change! Chien is Yang and Kun

Figure 2–2. The sixty-fourth hexagram—Wei-Chi.

is Yin. When Yin and Yang are united in their character, the weak and the strong attain their substance" (translated by Chan, 1963).

It is also possible to interpret the trigrams and hexagrams much more concretely, as does Professor Wang Ming, a famous expert on Taoism and the history of Chinese philosophy, who asserts that the 31st hexagram, "Hsien," is a description of a young man petting with his girlfriend on a date.

It is interesting to compare Wang Ming's interpretation with the traditional one. The traditional interpretation, though containing many physical images, is both more abstract and more oriented to the traditional use of the trigrams and hexagrams for divination. Both the traditional text and Wang Ming's reinterpretation consist of line-by-line analysis of the symbol. According to Legge's translation (1963) of the traditional text:

> Hsien indicates that (on the fulfillment of the conditions implied in it), there will be free course and success. Its advantageousness will depend on being firm and correct, (as) in marrying a young lady. There will be good fortune.
>
> 1. The first line, divided, shows one moving his great toes.
>
> 2. The second line, divided, shows one moving the calves of his legs. There will be evil. If he abides (quiet in his place), there will be good fortune.
>
> 3. The third line, undivided, shows one moving his thighs, and keeping close hold of those whom he follows. Going forward (in this way) will cause regret.
>
> 4. The fourth line, undivided, shows that firm correctness which will lead to good fortune, and prevent all occasion for repentance. If its subject be unsettled in his movement, (only) his friends will follow his purpose.

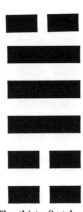

Figure 2–3. The thirty-first hexagram—Hsien.

5. The fifth line, undivided, shows one moving the flesh along the spine above the heart. There will be no occasion for repentance.

6. The sixth line, divided, shows one moving his jaws and tongue.

According to Professor Wang's new interpretation and translation (1982):

> Hsien kua indicates the intimacy between man and woman. The picture is woman above and man under her. If you get this kua, your wedding and marriage will be very good.
>
> 1. The first line, divided, represents the young man touching the girl's toes.
>
> 2. In the second line, divided, the young man gives her calves a heavy pinch; it is very painful and she pretends to escape. After the young man's sweet apologies, the girl agrees to stay with him. It is very nice.
>
> 3. In the third line, undivided, he touches her thighs lightly, and clasps her knees tightly, so that she cannot run away.
>
> 4. In the fourth line, undivided, she wants to leave because she is embarrassed that there are so many people passing by.
>
> 5. In the fifth line, undivided, he touches her neck between her mouth and heart. Their pleasure is intense.
>
> 6. In the sixth line, divided, he kisses her face, her mouth, and her tongue. (Translated by the author)

The most significant aspect of Wang Ming's reinterpretation is its implication that such a revered classic expresses an explicitly open and positive attitude toward sex.

The most important hexagram in terms of sexual symbolism may well be Number 63, called "Chi-Chi" (Completion), which is considered to symbolize sexual union. The upper trigram is Kan, which symbolizes "water," "clouds," and "woman," and the lower trigram is Li, which symbolizes "fire," "light," and "man." Through this combination, the hexagram expresses the perfect harmony of man and woman completing each other, graphically depicted by the perfect alternation of Yin and Yang lines (see Figure 2–4).

Achievement of this harmony was thought to be the basis of a happy and healthy sex life. Since the "Chi-Chi" trigram symbolized perfect sexual intercourse, one noted Taoist sexual handbook was entitled Chi-Chi-Chen-Ching (*True Manual of the "Perfected Equalization"*). (See Chapter 4.)

Many have said that one important result of the sexual revolution of the 1960s and 1970s was popularization of the "woman above" position in sexual intercourse. How interesting that in the *I-Ching*, which is more than 2,000 years old, the hexagram which places the symbol for man above the symbol for woman represents incompleteness and dis-

Figure 2–4. The sixty-third hexagram—Chi-Chi.

satisfaction, while the hexagram which places the symbol of woman above the symbol of man represents completion and satisfaction!

SEXUAL ATTITUDES IN THE CONFUCIAN, TAOIST, AND BUDDHIST TRADITIONS

In addition to ancestor worship and folk religion, there are three great literate traditions, generally known as the three religions of China. These include the teachings of the Confucian School (Rujia), Taoist teachings (Daojia, Taoism), and Buddhist teachings (Shijia). It is very important to analyze the attitudes toward sex in these three major cultural, philosophical, and religious traditions.

Confucianism

The chief literate tradition of China, Confucianism, is based on writings attributed to Confucius (Kongzi, or Master Kong, 551–479 B.C.), the first great educator, philosopher, and statesman of China, and his followers, especially Mencius (Mengzi, or Master Meng, 372–289 B.C.), a political thinker who believed in democracy.

There are two historic components of Confucianism: the earlier Rujia (Confucian school of philosophy) and the later Kongjiao (Confucian religion). The Rujia, which represents a political-philosophical tradition that was extremely important in early imperial times, is the element most directly connected with the persons and teachings of Confucius and Mencius—in fact, it is also known as "Kong Meng zhi dao" (the doctrine of Confucius and Mencius). The Kongjiao might best be described as the state's effort to fulfill the religious needs of the people within the framework of the Confucian tradition, an unsuccessful attempt which occurred in the late imperial period (A.D. 960–1911).

For some 2,000 years, Confucianism enjoyed almost unassailable prestige as the ideology of the imperial bureaucracy, and was essential to China's political unity. Regardless of how much a particular ruler might prefer Buddhism or Taoism, Confucianism had a role in the practical affairs of government which could not be denied or neglected. Philosophical Confucianism was very successful as a political ideology, as well as being an impressive system of moral philosophy.

Confucianism is frequently described as sex-negative, but that is incorrect. The Kongjiao of the late imperial period should not be taken as representative of Confucianism generally, and differs markedly from the preceding Rujia school. The least that can be said is that Confucianism's viewpoint on sex is not negative. Confucius himself never spoke slightingly of the sexual impulse.

Just as some of the earliest Western philosophical texts were lecture notes taken by students, the major record of Confucius' thought is the *Analects*, which consist of notes taken by his closest students. In the terminology of the *Analects*, something of which "the Master did not speak" was something of which he refused to speak because he disliked or opposed it. And, the *Analects* report, "The subjects on which the Master did not speak were extraordinary things, feats of strength, disorder, and spiritual being" (adapted from translation in Legge, 1971). Human sexuality is conspicuously missing from the list of subjects on which "the Master did not speak."

As noted earlier, the *I-Ching* contains several remarks of Confucius which imply a positive attitude toward sex, and the Confucian classics contain several comments which many Chinese are fond of quoting in support of people's sexual desires and rights. This might well surprise Western readers, since all too often the sexual implications of these aphorisms are literally lost in the translation. For example, the translations that follow had to be adapted from those of Legge (1983) because the original Chinese text contains the character "SE," which can mean "color," "beauty," or "sex," and Legge consistently avoids the third meaning, even when its use would make more sense. Thus, to give one example, he changes Gaozi's remark, "Eating food and having sex is human nature" to "To enjoy food and delight in colors is nature." Legge goes on to comment, on page 853, that "We might suppose that 'SE' here denoted 'the appetite of sex,' but another view is preferred." Without being told who prefers "another view" and why, it is all too easy to suspect that, as sometimes happens, the original Chinese has been refracted through a filter of Western prudery. The adaptations given here convey the true implications of Confucius' remarks.

According to the *Analects*, Book IX, Chapter 17, "The Master said, 'I have not seen one who loves virtue as he loves sex.' " This remark clearly implies that Confucius appreciated that the sexual impulse is integral to human nature, as did the comment in *The Book of Rites* (Li Ji), "Food and drink and the sexual relation between men and women compose the major human desires."

In *The Works of Mencius*, a major Confucian classic, Gaozi is quoted as saying, "Eating food and having sex is the nature of human beings." In addition, Mencius himself remarked, "To enjoy sex is the desire of human beings," and, "When teenagers and youths become conscious of sex, they will look toward young and beautiful women." A notably positive and permissive attitude was contained in a longer passage in which Mencius advocated the common people's right to sexual enjoyment:

> The king said, "I have an infirmity; I am fond of beauty and sex." The reply (by Mencius) was, "Formerly, King Tae was fond of beauty and sex, and loved his wife.... At that time, in the seclusion of the house, there were no dissatisfied women, and abroad, there were no unmarried men. If Your Majesty loves beauty and sex, let the people be able to gratify the same feeling, and what difficulty will there be in your attaining the imperial sway?"

The positive, permissive Confucian attitude toward sex was not unqualified. An important aspect of Confucian philosophy and ethics was a conception of ordered relationships as integral to a functioning society. The approbation given to sexual relationships, besides involving a belief that such relationships reflected an overarching natural order (the Yin-Yang concept), assumed a context of marriage and filial obligation. In the Confucian view, filial duty was a primary virtue, and the obligation to produce children was as important as the obligation to care for one's aged parents. It was in this context that Mencius could say:

> That male and female should dwell together, is the greatest of human relations. (Translated by Legge, 1983)

Taoism

Taoism, like Confucianism, has both a philosophical and a religious tradition. Like the Rujia and Kongjiao forms of Confucianism, the two streams of Taoism are markedly different. As with Confucianism, the philosophical system of Taoism developed earlier—it flourished early in the fifth century B.C., and the religion developed later—in the first century A.D. (about religious Taoism, see Chapter 4).

The Taoist philosophy is not one of quiet contemplation or idle speculation. It offers a practical way of life. However, some of its teachings were eventually incorporated into the mystical popular religion called "Daojiao." In China the religion and the philosophy are known to be separate, but in the West the similarity of their names has caused confusion, and both are known as "Taoism."

The origin of Taoist philosophy is obscure. The term "Tao" can be traced to the earliest Chinese classics, and it is a basic term in all ancient Chinese philosophical schools, including Confucianism. But it was in the work of Lao-tzu, author of the *Tao Te Ching*, that the Taoist philosophy developed.

Lao-tzu's book is so important to Chinese culture that one might well say that Chinese civilization, and the Chinese character, would have been utterly different if the *Tao Te Ching* had never been written. No one can hope to understand Chinese philosophy, religion, government, art, medicine, sexology—or even cooking—without a real appreciation of this profound philosophy. Taoism makes a unique contribution to Chinese life, for while Confucianism emphasizes social order and an active life, Taoism concentrates on individual life and tranquillity.

It is impressive that while the core of this philosophy is embodied in a small classic of about 5,250 Chinese characters, no other Chinese classic of such small size has exercised so much influence. More commentaries have been written on it than on any other Chinese classic: about 350 are extant, besides approximately 350 that are fragmentary or believed lost. The first translation of the *Tao Te Ching* into a Western language was a Latin translation made in A.D. 1788; since then, there have been translations into many foreign languages, which have been greatly influential for generations. Chan (1963) estimated that the *Tao Te Ching* has had more English translations than any other Chinese book, perhaps more than forty. By now, there may be over fifty.

The classic texts of both philosophical and religious Taoism express positive attitudes toward sex. The following quotes from the *Tao Te Ching* represent the approach of philosophical Taoism:

Chapter 6

The spirit of the valley never dies.
It is called the subtle and profound female.
The gate of the subtle and profound female
Is the root of Heaven and Earth.
It is continuous, and seems to be always existing.
Use it and you will never wear it out.

(Chan, 1963)

Chapter 42

The Tao gives birth to One.
One gives birth to Two.
Two gives birth to Three.
Three gives birth to all things.
All things have their backs to the female and stand facing male.
When male and female combine, all things achieve harmony.

(Mitchell, 1988)

Chapter 55

His bones are weak, his sinews tender, but his grasp is firm.
He does not yet know the union of male and female,
But his organ is aroused.
This means that his essence is at its height.

(Chan, 1963)

Chapter 61

The female by quiescence conquers the male;
By quiescence gets underneath.

(Waley, 1958)

The following quotations are from *The Canon of Peace and Tranquillity* (Taiping Jing), an early classic of religious Taoism.

Through the way of copulation between husband and wife, the Yin and Yang all obtain what they need and Heaven and Earth become peace and tranquillity.

Men and women are the roots of Yin and Yang....Let one man have two women, because Yang is odd numbers, and Yin is even numbers.

Based on one Yin and one Yang, Heaven allows both man and woman to exist and to be sexually attractive to each other, therefore life can be continued. (Wang Ming, 1960, translated by the author)

Another early classic of religious Taoism, *The Work of Ko Hung* (also known as Bao-pu-zi and by other titles—see Chapter 3), which was written in about A.D. 320, also displays a positive attitude toward sex. The passage quoted here emphasized the significance of sexual life for health, listing abstention from sexual intercourse as one of the several "wounds":

Someone observed: "Wouldn't you say that injury comes from lust and licentiousness?"

Pao Po Tzu replied: "Why only from that? The fundamental thing in macrobiotics is the reversion of one's years....If a man in the vigor of youth attains knowledge of how to revert his years (by the art of the bedchamber), absorbs the enchymona of the Yin to repair his brain, and gathers the Jade Juice from under the Long Valley, without taking any (prolongevity) drugs at all, he will not fail to live for three hundred years, though he may not become an immortal." (Adapted from translations in Ware, 1966, and Needham, 1983)

The religiously based belief that appropriate sexual behavior could contribute to health and even longevity led to the development of a variety of special techniques that will be discussed in Chapter 4, "Sexual Techniques of the Taoists: Myths and Methods."

Buddhism

Buddhism, the third great literate tradition in China, originated with the teachings of Gautama Buddha (565–486 B.C.) and traditions emanating from them. Missionaries carried these teachings out of India, and they developed into a world religion. From the time that Buddhism was first introduced into China in the first century A.D., its chief appeal lay in its promise of salvation. Buddhism offers to the Chinese people just what other religions offer to the people of other countries—something that comes to the rescue when human reason falters or seems to fail. Lin (1935) reported that Buddhist monks were more popular than Taoist monks and for every Taoist temple there were ten Buddhist temples. Buddhism has affected Chinese language and literature, and stimulated every aspect of the Chinese imagination. Buddhist monks and nuns were admitted into the privacy of the Chinese home as no other person was, being present at such important occasions as births, deaths, and weddings. Because of this special status, if one is to believe numerous Chinese novels, monks and nuns were indispensable to many a plot to seduce a widow or virgin.

Although most Buddhist schools abjured sexual desire, this teaching had little impact on the sexual attitudes of most Chinese people. Buddhist monks cannot marry, but most Chinese were not monks whether they believed in Buddhism or not. A "Jushi" (lay Buddhist) not only was permitted to marry but was even allowed to have several wives (one official wife and several concubines). To lay Buddhists, the injunction against salaciousness meant only that they should not have extramarital sex.

The Chinese people needed the services of the Buddhist clergy but were skeptical about their sexual purity. This attitude may have arisen from the belief, nurtured by the Taoist and Confucian traditions, that sexuality is deeply rooted in human nature. In any case, there were many sexual jokes, stories, and novels whose theme was that the Buddhist monks and nuns were quite interested in having sexual intercourse. Like the Catholic monks and nuns in the tales of Boccaccio, the Buddhist monks and nuns of Chinese fiction were frequently accused of outright immorality. One reason for this was that monks had unusual opportunities for contact with women who were not related to them. Confucian morality required the seclusion of women, who could only appear in public to visit the temples. Also, as noted earlier, monks could visit women in their homes for religious reasons. This unusual situation, coupled with a natural impulse to expose even a hint of hypocrisy, stimulated the production of fiction that was sometimes satiric, sometimes erotic, and sometimes even pornographic.

One of the more refined literary treatments of the sexual temptations of the Buddhist clergy is a poem called "A Young Nun's Worldly Desires." This particular treatment of a favorite literary subject is taken from a popular Chinese drama, "The White Fur Coat." It is a young nun's soliloquy:

> A young nun am I, sixteen years of age;
> My head was shaven in my young maidenhood.
> For my father, he loves the Buddhist sutras,
> And my mother, she loves the Buddhist priests.
> Morning and night, morning and night,
> I burn incense and I pray....
>
> When beauty is past and youth is lost,
> Who will marry an old crone?
> When beauty is faded and youth is jaded,
> Who will marry an old, shriveled cocoon?
> ...These candles of the altar,
> They are not for my bridal chamber.
> These long incense-containers,
> They are not for my bridal parlor.
> And the straw prayer cushions,
> They cannot serve as quilt or cover,
>   Oh, God!
>
> Whence comes this burning, suffocating ardor?
> Whence comes this strange, infernal, unearthly ardor?
> I'll tear these monkish robes!
> I'll bury all the Buddhist sutras;
> I'll drown the wooden fish,
> And leave all the monastic putras!
>
> I'll leave the drums,
> I'll leave the bells,
> And the chants,
> And the yells,

And all the interminable, exasperating, religious chatter!

I'll go downhill, and find me a young and handsome lover—
Let him scold me, beat me!
Kick or ill-treat me!
I will not become a buddha!
(Translated by Lin, 1935)

Far more extreme were the tales in a special collection of thirty-one sexual and pornographic stories about Buddhist monks and nuns called Shengni Niehai (alternately translated as *The Ocean of Iniquities of Monks and Nuns*, or *Monks and Nuns in a Sea of Sins*). In one of the tales, the author described a Buddhist monk who abused his power in order to deflower virgins before their wedding ceremonies and to cruelly rape any woman who attracted him. Then the author concludes:

Bloody wind and sad rain
Stirred up waves in the River Ganges,
Filthy dew and shameful clouds
Covered over the Buddhist realms....

If one is not bald [Buddhist monks shaved their heads], one can't be
    evil;
If one is not evil, one can't be bald.
More lewdly evil because his head is bald,
Why is it then
That the four classes of people
Still call the monks Buddhas
And revere them as great masters?
(Translated by Yang & Levy, 1971)

There is evidence that this suspicion of the Buddhist clergy existed not merely because the situation of the monks seemed an invitation to immorality but also because immoral behavior really did occur. In his formal studies of the history of prostitution in China, Wang Shunu (1934) included a special section on Buddhist and Taoist nuns. He pointed out that many nuns really resembled prostitutes and their temples brothels. This was not "temple prostitution" of the kind that was institutionalized in the ancient Mediterranean world. In those cases, prostitution was part of the worship of a god or goddess (usually a fertility deity), and any money involved was an accepted way of raising funds for the temple. Buddhist and Taoist nuns' prostitution was simply seen as corruption.

Some Buddhist sects really did engage in exotic sexual practices. The cult known in the West by its Tibetan name of Tantrayana, or Tantrism, is known in China as Mi-tsung. This sect, which flourished during the Yuan dynasty, especially during the reign of Kublai Khan (A.D. 1216–

1294), taught that the "Buddha nature" resided in the female generative organs and stressed the mystical importance of sexual union (Needham, 1956). A description of the kinds of practices resulting from this doctrine is contained in the "Biography of Ha-Ma" in *The History of the Yuan Dynasty*:

> He [i.e., Ha-ma, prime minister] also presented to the Emperor [i.e., Hui-tsung, A.D. 1333–1367] the Tibetan monk Ka-lin-chen, who was an expert in the secret (Tantric) ritual. That monk said to the Emperor: "Your Majesty rules over all in the Empire, and owns all riches within the four seas. But Your Majesty should not think of this life only. Man's life is brief, therefore this secret method of the Supreme Joy (that ensures longevity) should be practised." The Emperor thereupon practised this method, which is called "Discipline in Pairs." It is also called "yen-tieh-erh," and "secret." All these practices refer to the Art of the Bedchamber. The emperor then summoned Indian monks to direct those ceremonies, and conferred upon a Tibetan monk the title of Ta-yuan-kuo-shih ("Master of the Great Yuan Empire"). They all took girls of good families... for these disciplines and called that "to sacrifice" (kung-yang). Then the Emperor daily engaged in these practices, assembling for the purpose great numbers of women and girls, and found his joy only in this dissolute pleasure. He also selected a number from among his concubines and made them perform the dance of the Sixteen Dakini (Shih-liu-tien-mo, the Sixteen Heavenly Devils) and the Eight Males (pa-lang). [Van Gulik speculated that this "dance" really consisted of sexual intercourse by sixteen couples representing mythical figures.]...The brothers of the Emperor and those men who are called "Companions" all engaged in front of the Emperor in these lewd embraces, men and women being naked. The hall where these things took place was called Chieh-chi-wu-kai, which means in Chinese "Everything without obstacle." Ruler and statesmen thus displayed their lewdness, and the crowd of monks went in and out of the Palace, and were allowed to do anything they liked. (translated in van Gulik, 1961)

Clearly, there was some tension between the usual Buddhist ideal of sexual purity and the unusual sexual practices of Tantric Buddhism. There was also an apparent tension between the demands for propriety and procreation in the Confucian system. Nonetheless, it cannot be denied that the symbolic importance of sexual interaction in the Confucian, Taoist, and Buddhist systems, and the practical and ritual importance of reproduction, all contributed to positive attitudes toward human sexuality. These attitudes were evidenced not only in the great classics and the refined productions of poets and dramatists but also, as the next section shows, in the folk literature of the common people.

THE PEOPLE'S VOICE: LOVE AND SEX IN *SHE KING*

The *She King* (Shih Ching, Shi Jing), is the oldest repository of Chinese verse. It was probably first compiled in the early sixth century B.C., collecting 305 poems and folk songs dating from between the sixteenth and eleventh centuries B.C. to the sixth century B.C. Like the *I-Ching*, it is counted among the five Confucianist classics.

The existing Chinese edition of *She King*, was compiled, numbered, and annotated by the Han Dynasty scholar Maou Heng, and is appropriately called *Maou Shi (Maou's Book of Poetry)*. There are numerous English translations, including James Legge's the *She King* (subtitled *The Book of Poetry*, originally published in 1871 and reprinted in 1971), Arthur Waley's translation *The Book of Songs* (1937), and Bernard Kargren's *The Book of Odes* (1950).

Shi Ji (Historical Records) contains a memoir of Confucius by Ssuma Chhien (146–86 B.C.), in which he says:

> The old poems amounted to more than 3,000. Confucius removed those which were only repetitions of others, and selected those which would be serviceable for the inculcation of propriety and righteousness. Ascending as high as Seeh and How-tseih, and descending through the prosperous eras of Tin and Chow to the times of decadence under kings Yew and Le, he selected in all 305 pieces, which he sang over to his lute, to bring them into accordance with the musical style of the Shaou, the Woo, the Ya, and the Sung. (Translated in Legge, 1971)

This carefully edited collection by Confucius includes many poems about love and sex. In fact, the famous poem which is number one in Maou's edition is a love poem:

Kuan tseu (Number 1)

Kuan-kuan goes to the ospreys,
On the islet in the river.
The modest, retiring, virtuous, young lady—
For our gentleman a good mate she.
Here long, there short, is the duckweed,
To the left, to the right, borne about by the current
The modest, retiring, virtuous, young lady—
Waking and sleeping, he sought her.
He sought her and found her not,
And waking and sleeping he thought about her.
Long he thought; oh! long and anxiously;
On his side, on his back, he turned, and back again.
(Adapted by the author from Legge, 1971)

Some poems were more explicitly sexual, like the following:

Ya yew sze keun (Number 23)

Dead doe in the clearing
White reeds entangle it
Lady's bosom plump with spring
Bold gentleman who plays with her.

Tender young tree in the forest
Dead deer in the clearing
White reeds bind it
Lady like jade:
"Slowly and gently, O gently
O do not crumple my petticoat
Do not cause your hairy dog to bark."
(Translation adapted by the author from Scott, 1972)

In all, *She King* contains dozens of poems relating to love, sex, and marriage, many of them of great lyrical beauty. It is of crucial significance that Confucius, who edited *She King* with the avowed purpose of selecting poems that would inspire ethical behavior, retained these poems. They are proof that the founder of China's great ethical tradition shared his people's profound respect for human sexuality.

Chapter 3

"Inside the Bedchamber"
Classical Chinese Sexology

Thanks to the Yin-Yang philosophy and the positive sexual attitudes prevalent in ancient times, China is the source of the world's oldest sexological texts. When the Chinese began recording their sexual beliefs and knowledge is unknown. The oldest known texts, which were clearly based on an already well-developed tradition, were written more than 2,000 years ago.

As will be shown, these texts generally intertwine three themes: the mystical benefits of sexual intercourse, the health benefits of intercourse conducted according to certain theories, and the inherent pleasurability of sexual contact. Despite their burden of alchemical symbolism, many of these works are as remarkable for their acute naturalistic observation as for their sharp contrast with the prudery of many contemporary Western thinkers and of later eras in Chinese history.

THE EARLIEST CHINESE SEX BOOKS

The Oldest Known Texts

As noted in Chapter 1, excavations at Former Han Tomb No. 3 in Hunan province brought to light fourteen medical texts which had been buried in 168 B.C. Three of these books are sexological texts, titled by the discoverers *Ten Questions and Answers* (Shi-wan), *Methods of Intercourse between Yin and Yang* (He-yin-yang-fang), and *Lectures on the Super Tao in the World* (Tian-xia-zhi-tao-tan) (Li, Chen, & Ruan, 1987), the earliest extant Chinese sexological works. These ancient classics provided very explicit instructions regarding techniques of sexual intercourse. The following example is drawn from a section of *Lectures on the Super Tao in the World*, subtitled "Seven Injuries and Eight Advantages" (qi sun ba yi):

> Before coitus, you should engage in foreplay with her until she wants to be entered. This principle is called "zhi-shi," meaning that you must know what is the right time; in short, "wait until the right time."
>
> You should wait and let your penis become harder and larger. This principle is called "xu qi"—"accumulating your vital energy [chi]."
>
> You should insert it slowly and be in harmony with your lady. This principle is called "huo-mei"—"harmony with your woman."
>
> You may sometimes thrust strongly and rapidly, and sometimes keep your penis in her vagina without any movement at all, to wait and let her sexual climax come. This principle is called "dai-yin" (obtaining orgasm).
>
> After your ejaculation, you should withdraw when your penis is still half-erect. This principle is called "ding-qing" (getting out/ leaving at the right time). (Yi Jiancun, 1980; Zhou Yimiu, 1989; translated by the author)

The concept of the "Seven Injuries and Eight Advantages" was an important element of classical Chinese sexology and traditional Chinese medicine, which was also emphasized in the Yellow Emperor's Canon of Medicine, mentioned in the previous chapter as the oldest and greatest medical classic extant in China. The book consists of two sections, the *Plain Questions* (Su Wen), written in the form of a dialogue, and the *Miraculous Pivot*, also known as the *Canon of Acupuncture* (Ling Shu). The questions cover a great variety of subjects, including the relationship between humanity and nature, the medical application of the theories of Yin and Yang and of the Five Elements, the theory of the promotion of the flow of vital energy, and specific discussions of human anatomy and physiology, etiology of diseases, pathology, diagnosis and treatment, disease prevention, and health maintenance generally. The concept of the "Seven Injuries and Eight Advantages" was particularly emphasized in the following passage:

> Chi Po answered: "...Thus Yin and Yang alternate, their victories vary and so does the character of their diseases."
>
> The Yellow Emperor asked: "Can anything be done to blend and to adjust these two principles in nature?"
>
> Po answered: "If one has the ability to know the seven injuries and the eight advantages, the two principles can be brought into

harmony. If one does not know how to use this knowledge then his span of life will be limited by early decay...." (Veith, 1972)

This passage exemplifies the difficulty of translating the ancient Chinese medical texts. Veith's literal translation of the four Chinese characters "qi sun ba yi" into the phrase "(the) seven injuries (and the) eight advantages" without any explanation is correct, while that of Lu (1978), a traditional Chinese medical expert who translated "qi sun ba yi" by explaining it as "menstruation in women and growth of sex energy in men," was incorrect. Lu's error is understandable because, before the discovery of the manuscript of *Lectures on the Super Tao in the World*, no one could know the meaning of the ancient phrase "qi sun ba yi."

An example of the detailed descriptions of sexual response and techniques to be found in the ancient sexological works is the following excerpt from *Methods of Intercourse between Yin and Yang:*

> The methods of union of female and male (Yin and Yang) in sexual intercourse are as follows. The man starts by touching and stroking the Yang (back) side of her wrist, then along both sides of her forearm and elbow, reaching into her underarm. Continuously, he slips his hand around and passes the top of her shoulder, moving up into the nape of her neck. Then he touches and massages her "Chengguang" point [located at the center of the nape of the neck], around to the front of her neck moving in a circle, and down to her "Quepen" point [located in the midpoint of the supraclavicular fossa]. Continuing downward he touches her nipple, he fondles the soft flesh around her breasts, and moves down between her breasts. Finally, he comes to the bottom of her abdomen around her pubic bone. He reaches her vagina and touches the clitoris. In this manner the man absorbs the natural vital energy [chi] and invigorates his mind and spirit. Therefore, the man will attain to longevity in harmony with the heaven and earth.

The text goes on to assert that touching and fondling the clitoris with a down-to-up motion gives physical comfort to the woman's entire body, as well as mental stimulation and emotional satisfaction. It adds that foreplay, kissing, and embracing can arouse strong passions even without a consummation of the sexual act, then outlines certain principles and methods of foreplay.

> *One:* When the vital energy [chi] moves upward, and the face is suffused with warmth, you should let your breathing slow down.
> *Two:* When her nipples firm up and beads of sweat appear on her nose, you embrace her slowly.
> *Three:* When the coating on her tongue looks light and thin, and the surface of the tongue looks smooth, you two should kiss each other and keep mutual submission.

Four: When her vaginal secretion flows out and moistens her legs, you should strike her vulva with your penis.

Five: When she begins repeatedly swishing her tongue and swallowing, you should gently sway her body.

These are the five signals of female sexual arousal. When all the five signals of arousal have occurred, it is time to move on from foreplay into sexual intercourse. (Zhou Yimiu, 1989; translated by the author)

Earliest Bibliographies and Essays Concerning Sexology

Pan Ku (Ban Gu, A.D. 32–92), one of China's greatest historians, was the chief official historian during the reign of Emperor Ming Ti (A.D. 57–75) of the Later Han Empire. Pan Ku was the major author of *The History of the Former Han Dynasty from 206 B.C. to A.D. 23* (Han Shu). This work includes a section entitled "Bibliography of Literary Works" (Yi-Wen-Zhi), which lists the titles of the most important books then available, classified according to content. Pan Ku included a special heading for "fang zhong" (literally "inside the bedchamber," and usually translated as "the art of the bedchamber," "the art of the bedroom," or sometimes directly as "the sexual techniques"). Fang zhong were listed immediately after medical works. This list of eight works included annotations, reproduced here, stating how many "juan" comprised each book. A juan was a scroll (of paper or silk), usually containing a chapter or major segment of a work. It is usually translated as "roll" or "volume." Pan Ku's list is given in Table 3–1.

Pan Ku concluded his list of fang zhong with a commentary which is the earliest extant essay on Chinese sexology:

Table 3–1. Books Concerning the Art of the Bedchamber Contained in *History of the Former Han Dynasty*

Jung-ch'eng-yin-tao	*Sex Handbook of Master Jung-Ch'eng*	26 rolls
Wu-Ch'eng-tzu-yin-tao	*Sex Handbook of Master Wu-Ch'eng*	36 rolls
Yao-shun-yin-tao	*Sex Handbook of the Emperors Yao and Shun*	23 rolls
T'ang-pan-keng-yin-tao	*Sex Handbook of the Kings T'ang and Pan Keng*	20 rolls
T'ien-lao-tsa-tzu-yin-tao	*Sex Handbook of T'ien Lao and Others*	25 rolls
T'ien-yi-yin-tao	*Sex Handbook of T'ien-yi*	24 rolls
Huang-ti-san-wang-yang-yang-fang	*Recipes for Nursing Potency by Yellow Emperor and Three Kings*	20 rolls
San-chia-nei-fang-yu-tzu-fang	*Recipes for the Bedchamber and the Obtaining of Offspring of the Three Schools*	17 rolls

The Art of the Bedchamber constitutes the climax of human emotions, it encompasses the Super Tao. Therefore the Saint Kings of an-
tiquity regulated man's outer pleasures in order to restrain his inner
passions and made detailed rules for sexual intercourse. A familiar
quotation says: "The ancient Kings created sexual pleasure thereby
to regulate all human affairs." If one regulates his sexual pleasure he
will feel at peace and attain a high age. If, on the other hand, one
abandons himself to its pleasure, disregarding the rules set forth in
the above-mentioned treatises, one will fall ill and harm one's very
life. (Ban Gu, 1983; translated by van Gulik, 1961)

Pan Ku's work demonstrates that more than 2,000 years ago, sexology was not only a well-developed academic field but also a respected
subject of inquiry.

Unfortunately, all the books Pan Ku listed were lost in the many
wars and repeated book burnings that have marred China's history. Our
current knowledge of these works is derived entirely from references and
quotations in other surviving texts.

One such reference is contained in the poem "Tung-shen-ko," written by Chang Heng, one of ancient China's most eminent scientists and
poets. Chang Heng (A.D. 73–139) invented the oldest known astronom-
ical device and earthquake-measurement apparatus and originated the
"Hun Tien (ecliptic) theory." He was the chief official astronomer during the reigns of Emperor An Ti (A.D. 106–125) and Emperor Shun Ti
(A.D. 125–145). He also was a celebrated writer. In Tung-shen-ko, one of
his famous poems, a bride speaks to her husband in anticipation of the
joys of their wedding night:

> ...I have swept clean the pillow and the bedmat,
> And I have filled the burner with rare incense.
> Let us now lock the double door with its golden lock,
> And light the lamp to fill our room with its brilliance.
> I shed my robes and remove my paint and powder,
> And roll out the picture scroll by the pillow's side.
> The Plain Girl (Immaculate Girl) I shall take as my instructress,
> So that we can practice all the variegated postures,
> Those that an ordinary husband has but rarely seen,
> Such as taught by T'ien-lao to the Yellow Emperor.
> No joy shall equal the delights of this first night.
> These shall never be forgotten, however old we may grow.
>   (Translated by van Gulik, 1961)

From this poem we can learn several important points. (1) Chang's
reference to T'ien-lao verifies Pan Ku's listing of *T'ien-lao-tsa-tzu-yin-tao*
as one of the eight important sexological books in his time. (2) The poem
verifies that painted illustrations of sexual positions and the book *Canon*

of the Immaculate Girl (Su Nu Ching), of which portions are still extant, were already available at least before A.D. 139. (3) The poem demonstrates the period's positive valuation not only of sexuality but also of sex education. A government official freely and vividly describing the sexual relationship, explicit illustrations of sexual intercourse for the instruction of married couples, and a young bride expressing her desire for her husband without shame or fear would all be impossible in China today. The poem, whose publication would now be prohibited, is evidence of a heritage denied.

Another passage referring to a sex book listed by Pan Ku occurs in a poetical essay by the Han scholar Pian Jang (?–A.D. 200). This essay describes the delights of visiting dancing girls. The text was preserved in Pian Jang's biography in *History of the Later Han Dynasty, A.D. 25–220* (Hou Han Shu). Having described the dancing itself, Pian goes on to describe the pleasure of the dancers' company:

> He retires to a spacious tower, cooled by the breeze, and there practises the important methods of the Yellow Emperor. He takes the tender hand of a girl beautiful like Hsi-shih [a famous beauty in ancient China], and the white arm of another one like Mao-shih [another literary paragon of beauty]. Their bodies are beautiful, supple like grass moving in the wind, they put forth all their charms so that one forgets life and death. Then, when the bright morning dawns, ... (Translated by van Gulik, 1961)

The text in which this passage is quoted includes a brief comment explaining that the "methods of the Yellow Emperor" included such sexual techniques as suppression of ejaculation meant to increase longevity (see Chapter 4).

Later Bibliographies of Sexological Texts

The second dynastic history that listed sexological works was the *History of the Sui Dynasty, A.D. 581–617* (Sui Shu), edited primarily by Wei Zheng (A.D. 581–643), who was a famous Tang dynasty prime minister. Unlike Pan Ku, Wei Zheng did not devote a special category to fang zhong. Instead, he concluded the section on "Medical Books" by listing the titles of several sex handbooks. This listing is given in Table 3–2, which is based on Wei Zheng (1973) and van Gulik (1961).

The original texts of these books have also been lost. Fortunately, however, some long fragments of the first three and a few passages from the eighth have been preserved in Japanese collections. This material will be discussed in a section devoted to research on Japanese collections of Chinese texts.

Table 3–2. Sex Handbooks Included among "Medical Books" in *History of the Sui Dynasty*

Su-nu-pi-tao-ching	*Classic of the Secret Methods of the Plain Girl*	1 book roll
Hsuan-nu-ching	*Handbook of Sex of the Dark Girl*	1 book roll
Su Nu Fang	*Recipes of the Plain Girl*	1 book roll
Yu-fang-pi-chueh	*Secret Prescription for the Bedchamber*	8 book rolls
Hsin-Chuan-yu-fang-pi-chueh	*New Revised Secret Presciption for the Bedchamber*	9 book rolls
Hsu T'ai-shan: Fang-nei-pi-yao	*Summary of the Secrets of the Bedchamber,* by Hsu T'ai-shan	1 book roll
Hsu-fang-nei-pi-shu	*An Introduction to the Secret Art of the Bechamber,* by Mr. Ko	1 book roll
P'eng-tsu-yang-hsing	*P'eng-tsu on Nurturing Nature*	1 book roll
Yang-sheng-yao-chi	*Principles of Nurturing Life,* by Chang Chan	10 rolls

Other portions of these works are contained in some later Chinese histories. The *Old History of the Tang Dynasty, A.D. 618–906* (Chiu Tang Shu), edited by Liu Hsu in A.D. 945 (see Liu Hsu, 1975), contains *The Secret Art of the Bedchamber,* by Mr. Ko, in one book roll, and *Secret Prescription for the Bedchamber,* by Chung-huo-zi, in eight book rolls (Liu Hsu, 1975).

The *New History of the Tang Dynasty, A.D. 618–906* (Hsin Tang Shu), edited by Ouyang Hsiu and Sung Chhiin A.D. 1061 (see Ouyang & Sung, 1975), contains the same books with only a slight bibliographical difference, describing *Secret Prescription for the Bedchamber* as consisting of ten book rolls.

It should be noted that in later dynastic histories, such as the *History of the Sung Dynasty, A.D. 960–1279,* edited by Tho-Tho and Ouyang Hsuan in A.D. 1345, and the History of the Ming Dynasty, A.D. 1368–1643, edited by Chang Thing-yu and others from A.D. 1646 to 1736, no further reference is made to any sexological texts. These omissions might mean that the books in question had already been lost, or that later historians felt that they should not include such books in formal histories (or both).

RELATIONSHIPS AMONG MEDICAL, TAOIST, AND SEXOLOGICAL BELIEFS AND WRITINGS

Traditional Chinese medicine, Taoist sexual techniques, and classical sexology shared a common foundation in the principles of Yin and Yang, the five elements, and the concept of chi (vital energy). Thus, in addition to sharing content and terminology, they were consistent in their positive approach to sexuality. The most famous experts, Ge Hong, Tao Hongjing, and Sun Simiao, combined the roles of physician, Taoist master, and sexologist. Scholars such as these all stressed the value of a satisfactory sex life; this attitude, and the intermingling of the three academic disciplines, are illustrated in the following excerpts, which are given in chronological order.

Wei Po-yang's Tsan-tung-chi

Textual Research on the Taoistic and Magical Interpretation of the Book of Changes (Chou-i-tsan-tung-chi, often abbreviated as Tsan-tung-chi), consisting of 90 paragraphs, is said to have been written in about A.D. 150 by the famous Taoist adept Wei Po-yang. In this essay the extraction of mercury from cinnabar and lead is discussed in parallel with the sexual act, and against a metaphysical background of the theory of the Five Elements and of the symbolism of the *I-Ching*. Thus an accurate translation of much of Tsan-tung-chi must convey two or three levels of meaning—the alchemical, the sexual, and, often, the cosmological. The following excerpt of a translation by van Gulik (1961) is an example of this type of multiple translation:

> Ch'ien (the man) moves and is strong, his chi (vital energy) spreads out and his semen is stirred. K'un (the woman) remains still and harmonious, she constitutes (her womb) a haven for Tao (i.e., the process of procreation). When "hard" (penis) has shed (its semen), "soft" (vagina) dissolves into moisture. Nine times returning, seven times resuming, eight times coming back, six times remaining (inside).
>
> "Hard" and "soft" remain apart. The spending of seed (of Heaven, and the man), and the giving shape to that seed (by Earth, and the woman), is the natural way of Heaven and Earth, is as natural as a fire when started blazing upward, and running water flowing downward.

Ge Hong's Bao-pu-zi

Ge Hong (or Ko Hung, A.D. 281–341), also known as Ge (or Ko) Zhi-Chuan and Bao Pu Zi (Pao P'u Tzu), was a renowned physician and alchemist. He is best known as the author of *The Work of Ko Hung* (variously rendered as Bao-pu-zi, Pao Po Tzu, or Pao-pu-tzu), a treatise on alchemy, dietetics, and some magical practices, and of *A Handbook of Prescriptions for Emergencies* (Zhou Hou Bei Ji Fang).

The extant reprint of Bao-pu-zi consists of three parts—Nei Pian, Wai Pian, and an appendix. Nei Pian, "The Inner Collections," translated by James R. Ware (1966), includes several important paragraphs on sexual techniques, including a passage already discussed in the section on Taoism in Chapter 2, and others that are so important to an understanding of the relationship between certain Taoist ideas and traditional Chinese sexual theory and practice that they are quoted at length here. (The author used the conventional dialogue form.)

> INTERLOCUTOR: I have been taught that he who can fully carry out the correct sexual procedures can travel alone and summon gods and genii. Further, he can shift disaster from himself and absolve his misdeeds; turn misfortune into good; rise high if in office; double his profits if in business. Is it true?
>
> KO: This is all deceptive, exaggerated talk found in the writings of mediums and shamans....
>
> The best of the sexual recipes can cure the lesser illnesses, and those of a lower quality can prevent us from becoming empty; but that is all. There are very natural limits to what such recipes can accomplish. How could they ever be expected to confer the ability to summon gods and genii and to dispel misfortune or bring good?
>
> It is inadmissible that man should sit and bring illness and anxieties upon himself by not engaging in sexual intercourse. But then again, if he wishes to indulge his lusts and cannot moderate his dispersals, he hacks away at his very life. Those knowing how to operate the sexual recipes can check ejaculation, thereby repairing the brain; revert their sperm to the Vermilion Intestine...gather saliva into the Pool of Gold (? gall bladder)...conduct the three southern and the five northern breaths to their Flowered Rafters (? lungs). They can thus cause a man, even in old age, to have an excellent complexion, and terminate the full number of his allotted years.
>
> The crowd, however, learning that the Yellow Emperor mounted to heaven after having a harem of 1200, proceeds to claim that this was the sole reason he attained Fullness of Life. They do not know that...his success was not due to that sole fact.
>
> In sum, there is no benefit from taking all sorts of medicine and eating beef, mutton, and pork, if one does not know the arts of sexual intercourse. The Ancients, therefore, fearing that people might treat existence itself lightly or arbitrarily, purposely lauded these arts beyond complete credibility. Sexual intercourse may be compared with water and fire, either of which can slay man or bring him life, depending solely upon his ability to deal with them. On the whole, if the important rules are known, the benefits will be proportionate to the number of one's successive copulations. If, however, the procedure is employed in ignorance, sudden death could ensue after only

one or two copulations. Old P'eng's methods contain all the essentials. Other books on the subject teach only many troublesome methods difficult to carry out, and the resulting benefits are not necessarily as claimed. Man is scarcely able to follow the directions, and there are thousands of words of oral directions. Whoever does not know them would still be unable to attain Fullness of Life, even though he took many medicines. (Translated by Ware, 1966)

From these paragraphs we can see that Taoists and traditional Chinese medical doctors emphasized the significance of sex to health and longevity. Perhaps the most fascinating aspect of the discourse is that, although it makes claims we know to be untrue, it also offers a skeptical explanation of the still more fantastic claims that abounded at the time. No doubt the rejection of other claims gave these procedures the appearance of credibility.

Tao Hongjing's Yang Hsing Yen Ming Lu

On Delaying Destiny by Nourishing the Natural Forces (Yang Hsing Yen Ming Lu), also known by the alternate title *Achieving Longevity and Immortality by Regaining the Vitality of Youth* (Yang Sheng Yen Ming Lu), was a Taoist classic generally attributed to Tao Hongjing.

Tao Hongjing (A.D. 452–536) was a native of Danyang, now Nanjing of Jiangsu province, who specialized in studying the medicinal uses of herbs. He compiled *Commentary on Sheng Nong's Herbal* (Ban Cao Jing Ji Zhu), one of the most valuable early materia medica in China, describing 730 varieties of medical substances derived from vegetable, animal, and mineral sources.

The sixth chapter of *Delaying Destiny,* titled "On the Harms and Benefits of Having Sex with Women," is devoted to a sexual regimen.

> Changing of partners can lead to longevity and immortality. If a man unites with one woman only, the Yin chi [vital energy] is feeble and the benefit small. For the Tao of the Yang is modelled on Fire, that of the Yin on Water, and Water can subdue Fire, the Yin can disperse the Yang, and use it unceasingly...so that the latter becomes depleted, and instead of assistance to the repair and regeneration (of the Body) this is loss. But if a man can couple with twenty women and yet have no emission, he will be fit and of perfect complexion when in old age.... When the store of ching [reproductive essence] sinks low, illnesses come, and when it is altogether used up, death follows. (Li & Shen, 1987; Sun, 1982; translated by Needham, 1983)

Sun Simiao's Qian Jin Fang

Sun Simiao (A.D. 581–682), a native of Huayuan, now Yao County, Shanxi Province, was a famous Taoist, a prominent physician, and the author of *Prescriptions Worth a Thousand Pieces of Gold for Emergencies* (Bei Ji Qian Jin Yao Fang), written in A.D. 652, and the *Supplement to Prescriptions Worth a Thousand Gold Pieces* (Qian Jin Yi Fang), written in A.D. 682. These two books were prized as the first Chinese clinical medical encyclopedia and a compilation of the medical achievements preceding the seventh century.

Much of the sexological material in *Prescriptions* is virtually identical, even in language, with the material in *On Delaying Destiny*, as can be seen from the brief excerpt quoted here:

> The principle of the Art of the Bedchamber is very simple, yet few people can really practise it. The method is to copulate on one night with ten different women without emitting semen even a single time. This is the essence of the Art of the Bedchamber. (Sun Simiao, 1982; translated by van Gulik, 1961)

MATERIALS PRESERVED IN JAPANESE COLLECTIONS

From the fifth to nineteenth centuries A.D., Japan absorbed a great deal of Chinese culture, including medical knowledge; contact with Chinese culture was most intense during China's Tang dynasty (A.D. 618–907). For example, in Japan in A.D. 984 there were 204 Chinese medical books which were to be found in China during the Sui (A.D. 581–618) and Tang dynasties (Li, Cheng, & Ruan, 1987).

In the years from A.D. 982 to 984, the famous Japanese physician Tamba Yasuyori (A.D. 912–995) edited a voluminous compendium of medical science called in Japanese *I-shim-po* (in Chinese, Yi Xin Fang or I-hsin-fang), *The Essence of Medical Prescriptions*. Yasuyori, who was of Chinese descent (and, in fact, of noble lineage), was well suited to his task, and his treatise became a standard reference work for Japanese medical practitioners. Today it is the oldest medical monograph extant in Japan (Li, Cheng, & Ruan, 1987; Ishihara & Levy, 1968; Gulik, 1961). For many centuries this book existed only in manuscript form. Finally, in 1854, Taki Genkin (?–1857), a physician for the Shogun's harem, published a magnificent blockprint edition based on the best manuscripts.

The *I-shim-po* is an extremely valuable repository of ancient Chinese works, quoting more than 200 Han, Sui, and Tang sources, most of which are not available elsewhere. The only form in which many of these Chinese sources survive is in these quotations. Better yet, Yasuyori was such a conscientious scholar that he reproduced those passages he selected exactly as he found them in the original manuscripts brought over from China, not even correcting obvious errors, abbreviations, and repetitions.

Because Japanese orthography had not yet diverged from the Chinese at the time Yasuyori was working, his entire book is in the original Chinese, without any translations. Thus it is an excellent source for the rediscovery of lost Chinese medical works.

The twenty-eighth volume of this thirty-volume book is a special section on Chinese sexology, entitled "Fang Nei" (another way of saying "The Art of the Bedchamber"). This volume consists entirely of quotations culled from a number of ancient Chinese texts including sex manuals, medical treatises, books on physiognomy, collections of recipes, and so forth. The quotations were divided according to thirty subjects, listed in Table 3–3.

Under each subtitle, Yasuyori quoted several paragraphs from one or more of the following Chinese books: *Canon of the Immaculate Girl* (Su Nu Ching), *Prescriptions of the Immaculate Girl* (Su Nu Fang), *Important Matters of the Jade Chamber* (Yu Fang Chih Yao), *Secret Instructions Concerning the Jade Chamber* (Yu Fang Pi Chueh), *Book of the Mystery-Penetrating Master* (Tung Hsuan Tzu), *Prescriptions Worth a Thousand Pieces of Gold for Emergencies* (Bei Ji Qian Jin Yao Fang), and others. Since most of these works are preserved nowhere else, this text is of incalculable value.

THE AVAILABILITY OF ANCIENT SEXOLOGICAL WORKS IN MODERN CHINA

Though Yasuyori's work was based entirely on ancient Chinese sources, it was not discovered by Chinese scholars until 1870, when it was found by the scholar Yang Shou-ching, who had traveled to Japan for the express purpose of finding books which were lost in China. Another famous Chinese scholar, Yeh Te-hui, also came across the twenty-eighth chapter of *I-shim-po* in 1902 while doing research in the former Imperial Library at Ueno. Recognizing that it contained valuable Chinese sources no longer extant in their original form, he extracted these quotations and rearranged them according to the titles of the books from which they were originally drawn. The resulting compilation was published in 1903 as part of a larger compendium of rare Chinese sources. Yeh Te-hui's compilation was published as a series called the *Double Plum-Tree Collection* (Shuang-mei-ching-an-ts'ung-shu). The first volume of the series con-

Table 3–3. Yasuyori's Classification of Sexological Texts[a]

A. Sexual Philosophy

   1. Fundamental Principles
   2. Nourishing the Male Element
   3. Nourishing the Female Element

B. Sexual Arousal, Foreplay, and Sexual Responses

   4. Harmonizing the Will
   5. Controlling the Boudoir
   6. The Five Constancies
   7. The Five Signs
   8. The Five Desires
   9. The Ten Movements
  10. The Four Attainments

C. Sexual Techniques and Positions

  11. The Nine Essences
  12. The Nine Ways
  13. The Thirty Ways
  14. The Nine Styles
  15. The Six Postures

D. Sexual Hygiene and Medicine, and Sexual Myths

  16. The Eight Benefits
  17. The Seven Injuries
  18. Returning the Semen
  19. Curing Illnesses
  20. Seeking Children
  21. (Sexually) Good Women
  22. (Sexually) Evil Women
  23. Prohibitions
  24. Breaking Off Intercourse with Devils
  25. Making Use of Medicinal Properties
  26. Smallness of the Jade Stalk
  27. Largeness of the Jade Gate
  28. A Maiden's Pain
  29. An Older Woman's Injuries

[a]The author has categorized Yasuyori's subject headings.

sists of six sex booklets, five of which are reconstructions from *I-shim-po*. The contents of this volume are listed in Table 3–4.

The *Double Plum-Tree Collection* is a rare book in China now. Only a few major libraries have copies, and these—especially the first volume— are not available to the public. Yeh Te-hui himself, despite his distinguished reputation as one of the three most famous Confucian scholars of the early twentieth century, as a rare book collector, as a writer and publisher, and as a researcher in Chinese sexology, was killed in 1927 by Chinese

Table 3–4. Contents of First Volume of Shuang-mei-ching-an-tsung-shu
(Double Plum-Tree Collection), Edited and Annotated by Yeh Te-Hui

Chinese title	English title	Author/date
Su Nu Ching	Canon of the Immaculate Girl	Anonymous/Han dynasty
Su Nu Fang	Prescriptions of the Immaculate Girl	Anonymous/Han dynasty
Yu Fang Chih Yao	Important Matters of the Jade Chamber	Anonymous/Pre-Sui (before A.D. 581) perhaps fourth century
Yu Fang Pi Chueh	Secret Instructions Concerning the Jade Chamber	Anonymous/Pre-Sui (before A.D. 581) perhaps fourth century
Tung Hsuan Tzu	Book of the Mystery-Penetrating Master	Anonymous/Pre-Tang, perhaps fifth century
Thien Ti Yin Yang Ta Lo Fu[a]	Poetical Essay on the Supreme Joy	Pai Hsing-Chien (A.D. 775–82)

[a]This book was preserved in manuscript form only, in the monastic library of Tunhuang, until its recovery in our time (Needham, 1956).

Communist troops (*World Journal*, April 23, 30, June 13, 1987; *Centre Daily News*, April 23, 24, 1987; *The Young China Daily*, September 4, 1987).

Yasuyori's *I-shim-po* was reprinted in China in 1956. During the Cultural Revolution the publishers were severely criticized on behalf of the "revolutionary masses" because of the sexual content of the twenty-eighth volume of the book. An announcement was sent to libraries asking them to delete that portion of the book.

Thus, after the loss and rediscovery of these classics, a new censorship still denies the vast majority of Chinese people access to an important part of their heritage. Perhaps the best hope for making this information available lies with the Chinese presses outside mainland China. It was to increase the availability of some of this literature that the early issues of *Penthouse* (Chinese edition) published in Hong Kong in 1986 included reprints of *Su Nu Ching* (*Canon of the Immaculate Girl*) and other portions of Yeh's collection.

SOME HIGHLIGHTS OF THE CHINESE SEX CLASSICS

Both major sources described here have been translated into English—the twenty-eighth volume of *I-shim-po* was completely translated by Ishihara and Levy (1968), and the first volume of the *Double Plum-Tree Collection* was partially translated by van Gulik (1961). Moreover, parts of them were also translated by Chou (1971), Girchner (1957), and other authors. Since this material is available elsewhere, only some highlights will be given here.

Presumed Benefits of Intercourse for People of All Ages

All these works emphasize the importance of sexual life, even for the elderly. For example, both *On Delaying Destiny* and *Prescriptions* stress this point. Since, as noted previously, the same language is often used in both works, only one quotation (from *On Delaying Destiny*) is given here:

> The Chosen Girl asked Pheng Tsu, saying: "Ought a man sixty years of age to retain his ching (semen) entirely and guard it? Is it possible?"
>
> Pheng Tsu replied: "It is not. Man does not want to be without woman; if he has to do without her his mind will become restive, if his mind becomes restive his shen (spirit) will become fatigued, and his life-span will be shortened. Now if it were possible for him to keep his mind always serene, and untroubled by thoughts of sex, this would be excellent, but there is not one among ten thousand who can do it. If with force he tries to retain and block up (the semen), it will in fact be hard to conserve and easy to lose, so that it will escape (during sleep), the urine will become turbid, and he will suffer from the illness of haunting by incubi and succubi." (Chinese text, see Li & Shen, 1987; translated by Needham, 1983)

Instructions for Enjoyment of Intercourse

These classics were even more comprehensive than modern sex manuals. They offered detailed advice on the selection of sexual partners, flirting, and every aspect of coitus including foreplay, orgasm, and resolution. The following example is from *Secret Instructions Concerning the Jade Chamber*:

> [The Yellow Emperor asked,] "How can I become aware of the joyfulness of the woman?"
>
> Replied the Immaculate Girl: There are five signs, five desires, and ten movements. By looking at these changes you will become aware of what is happening in her body. The first of the five signs is called "reddened face"; if you see this you slowly unite with her. The second is called "breasts hard and nose perspiring"; then slowly insert the jade stalk [penis]. The third is called "throat dry and saliva blocked"; then slowly agitate her. The fourth is called "slippery vagina"; then slowly go in more deeply. The fifth is called "the genitals transmit fluid" [female ejaculation]; then slowly withdraw from her.

...The Immaculate Girl said: "Through the five desires, one is made aware of the woman's response, or what she wants you to do to her. First, if she catches her breath, it means that she wants to make love with you. Second, if her nose and mouth are dilated, it means that she wants you to insert your penis. Third, if she embraces you tightly, it means that she is very stimulated and excited. Fourth, if her perspiration flows and dampens her dress, it means that she wants to have her orgasm soon. Fifth, if her body straightens and her eyes close, it means she has already been satisfied. (Author's translation from Yasuyori, 1956)

As van Gulik (1961) has noted, the "five signs" correspond closely to the results of Kinsey's (1953) research. Despite some of the rather fanciful techniques prescribed for attaining longevity, the information on the sexual response does credit to the ancients' powers of observation.

Positions for Sexual Intercourse

The ancient Chinese were familiar with numerous positions for sexual intercourse: thirty are listed in *Book of the Mystery-Penetrating Master* (Tung Hsuan Tzu), nine in *The Classic of the Woman Profound* (Xian Nu Jing) (a lost book partially preserved in *I-shim-po*), and fifteen in *Secret Instructions Concerning the Jade Chamber* (Yu Fang Pi Chueh). The positions described in *Secret Instructions* are all supposed to have medical value. Although their translations are not entirely correct, all of these descriptions have been translated into English by Ishihara and Levy (1968) and others, and only a few examples are given here, translated by the author of this book:

The Mystery-Penetrating Master said: A careful investigation of postures of sexual intercourse has shown that there are but thirty main positions for consummating the sexual union. Among them there are flexing or extending; looking down or up; going out or in; being shallow or deep. With the exception of minor details these various positions and diverse movements are fundamentally the same and can be said to encompass all possibilities. I shall take them up one and all, model their postures, and record their special names which were given based on their pictorial images. The understanding reader will be able to probe their wonderful meaning to its very depth.

• • • • •

11. Sky-Soaring Butterfly
The man lies on his back and opens his legs wide. The woman sits lightly on his thighs, face-to-face, resting her weight on her two

feet on the bed. Then with her hands she guides his penis into her vagina.

12. *Reversed Flying Widgeon*

The man lies on his back face upward and opens his legs wide. The woman sits lightly on his thighs, back to face, resting her weight on her two feet on the bed. She lowers her head, embraces the man's penis, and inserts it into her vagina.

15. *The Paired Dance of the Female Blue Phoenixes*

[This passage of the ancient manuscript may include an erroneous Chinese character, so it is not clear. It is open to at least two different interpretations:]

(1) [A man and two women play together.] One woman lying on her back, and the other woman lying on her stomach. The one on her back raises her legs, the one on her stomach rides on top. Their two vaginas face one another. The man sits cross-legged, using his penis by inserting it in the vaginas above and below, thrusting upward and downward. [The author prefers this interpretation.]

(2) The woman lies face upward with her knees bent. The man squats over her with his penis in the vicinity of her vagina. He pushes his penis into her, thrusting upward and downward.

28. *The Cat and the Mouse Sharing One Cave*

[This passage of the ancient manuscript is unclear. It is open to at least two different interpretations:]

(1) [Two men and one woman play together.] The first man lies on his back and stretches his legs, the woman rides on top over his thighs, and he inserts his penis into her deeply. At the same time, another man lies on his stomach over her back, and inserts his penis into her vagina also.

[The author believes that the preceding is the correct interpretation, because in the Chinese text the characters "yiu nan" may be translated as "another man" instead of "another way, the man," and because the title "The Cat and the Mouse Sharing One Cave" could explicitly refer to two men (one cat, one mouse) sharing one woman. Other translators of this passage (Chang, 1977; Chou, 1971; Girchner, 1957; Humana & Wu, 1984; and Ishihara & Levy, 1968) have all translated it as a description of one man and one woman using two different postures, as in the example that follows. It is unlikely that the texts would describe two postures under one title. Perhaps the other translators believe that in ancient China there was no way two men could share one woman. However, it is not at all unlikely that such a menage à trois would take place, given the sex-positive attitudes

prevalent in ancient China. Indeed, the special significance of this
passage is that it provides evidence that such acts took place.]
    (2) The man lying on his back stretches his legs. The woman
lies above him and lets his penis enter deep inside her. Then the man
makes her lie on her stomach and rises to get on top of her, pushing
his penis into her.

Taoist Sexual Techniques

The texts described here provided the foundation for the development of Taoist sexual techniques, especially the methods suggested for
men to satisfy women, and to delay or avoid ejaculation. These later
developments are discussed in detail in Chapter 4.

Sexual Hygiene and Medicine

Because the disciplines of medicine and sexology were closely related, the discussion of sexuality included detailed recipes for herbal medicines thought to maintain general health, longevity, fertility, and potency.
For example, a combination of powdered deer-horn and aconite root is
prescribed for maintaining strength, youthfulness, potency, and a healthy
complexion. Another prescription is a combination of five ingredients,
to be taken with rice wine three times a day, as a cure for impotence,
accompanied by the claim that "A Governor of Shu Commandery (in
Szechwan) got a child when he was over seventy (through using this
prescription)" (translated by Ishihara & Levy, 1968).

THE ENDURING VALUE OF THE ANCIENT SEXOLOGICAL LITERATURE

Although much of the writing of the ancient sexologists has been
lost, their work has continued to have an effect on Chinese life and
thought. The work of later centuries, which will be described in detail
in subsequent chapters, rested on the ancient foundations. Even what
was known to be lost inspired the curiosity and imaginative effort of
later generations.
    In modern China, sadly, the value of this work is controversial. Yet
it is reasonable to hope that in time the respect that foreign scholars feel

for this work will encourage its appreciation in its native land, and support those scholars who seek to give it new life. Ultimately, this literature may contribute to China's renewal. Its celebration of sexual pleasure, and its emphasis on the need for enjoyment by both men and women, can be useful to the projects of sex education and women's liberation that are so crucial to modernization.

Sexual Techniques of the Taoists
Myths and Methods

THE ROLE OF TAOISM IN CHINESE CULTURE

Taoism is China's only genuine indigenous religion. Buddhism, a religion which certainly has been influential in Chinese culture, was imported from India. Confucianism, the other major indigenous system of thought, is secular in orientation, concerning itself with politics and ethics rather than the supernatural. Taoism, by contrast, possesses an herbal lore including medicines and aphrodisiacs; a cosmogony based on the principles of Yin and Yang and the five elements (metal, wood, water, fire, and earth); systems of magic, witchcraft, and astrology; a pantheon; a priesthood; and all the accompanying folklore. Thus, as noted Chinese scholar Lin Yutang remarked, "Taoism...accounts for a side of the Chinese character which Confucianism cannot satisfy...[offering] all those paraphernalia that go to make up a good, solid popular religion.... [It] was...the Chinese attempt to discover the mysteries of nature" (Lin, 1935).

While other religions have used sexual rites in connection with fertility cults, Taoism is one of the few that has stressed the importance of using sexual techniques for individual benefit. Unlike Tantric Hinduism, in which sexual ceremonies are meant to contribute to spiritual welfare, Taoist doctrine holds that appropriate sexual methods are a means of achieving personal immortality.

These sexual techniques have aroused considerable curiosity among foreigners, and fascinate Westerners because of their striking contrast with Western ascetic religions. Thus Tannahill (1980) comments:

While the Fathers of the early Christian church advocated sexual abstinence as the only sure route to heaven, other equally devout men in another part of the world took precisely the opposite view. "The more women with whom a man has intercourse, the greater will be the benefit he derives from the act," said one, and another added, "If in one night he can have intercourse with more than ten women it is best."

THE ROLE OF SEXUAL LORE IN TAOISM

The Broader Background of Taoist Sexual Mysticism

The exoticism of Taoist sexuality may have given Westerners an exaggerated idea of its religious importance. It should be remembered that these techniques were part of a larger system of physical hygiene whose most important technique was deep breathing. The central concept of this system was "chi," which may be translated as "vital energy." The concept of chi was almost universal in its application, being used in understanding celestial bodies and as the basis of martial arts and acupuncture therapy.

Those who used sexual practices to manipulate chi in the hope of one day being carried to heaven on the back of a stork were simply engaged in one aspect of a larger mystical system. Specifically, sexual techniques were referred to as "fang shu," "fang zhong," or "fang zhong shu." All three phrases have essentially the same meaning; literally "inside the bedchamber," more commonly translated as "the art of the bedchamber," or sometimes more frankly translated as "sexual technique." Since all three phrases refer to the same sexual techniques, they will be used interchangeably.

The Taoist Sects

It is typical for major popular religions to develop numerous sects over the course of centuries, and Taoism was no exception. Not all these sects placed equal emphasis on mystical practices, and of those that did, not all emphasized sexual methods.

The historical founder of the Taoist religion was Chang Ling, a popular religious leader and rebel. He urged his followers to read the *Tao-te ching* and in A.D. 143 organized them into "The Way of Five Dou of Rice," so named because Chang collected that amount of grain from members (a "dou" is a Chinese unit of dry measurement equivalent to ten liters). His followers called him "Heavenly Teacher" (Tien Shih), and he was the first in a succession of spiritual leaders. The last such leader, the sixty-third Celestial Master, Chang En-pu, fled from mainland China to Taiwan in 1949, and died there in 1969.

Eventually two major schools of Taoism developed. The first, or "Southern School," also known as the "Orthodox Unity School" (Zheng Yi Pai), or "The Way of the Heavenly Teacher" (Tien Shih Tao), was a highly organized religion. Followers of this school believed in a great number of gods of every description and many heroes and saints. It borrowed heavily from Buddhism, especially in its trinity of the Three Pure Ones, its belief in heavens and hells, and its clergy, monasticism, and canon. Its practices include temple worship, offerings to the dead, geomancy and other forms of divination, and the use of witchcraft and charms for driving away evil spirits and obtaining earthly blessings.

Followers of the other Taoist school, the "Northern School," also known as the "Perfect Realization School" (Quan Zhen Pai), sought immortality through meditation, breathing exercises, bathing, gymnastics, sexual arts, medicines, alchemy, and other means. These practices were partially codified by Wei Poyang in the second century A.D. Wei's *Textual Research on the Taoistic and Magical Interpretation of the Book of Changes* (Chou-i-tsan-tung-chi, sometimes abbreviated as Tsan-tung-chi, and referred to in Chapter 3) was an attempt to synthesize Taoist techniques for achieving immortality and the teachings of the occult *I-Ching (Book of Changes)*.

Later, the "Perfect Realization School" was further subdivided into two major branches: The older Southern Branch is also known as the "Ziyang Branch," after its Original Master, Ziyang Zhenren (also spelled Zhang Baiduan, or Chang Po-tuan) (984–1082). Ziyang Zhenren wrote the famous Taoist book *Understanding Reality: A Taoist Alchemical Classic* (Wu Chen Pien), translated into English by Thomas Cleary (1987); before the division into Northern and Southern Branches, it was a basic text of the Taoist philosophy, alchemical methodology, and sexual regimen. The Northern Branch, which for centuries had its headquarters at Beijing's White Cloud Monastery, was founded by Wang Chongyang (A.D. 1112–1170).

According to Zhang Mingcheng (1974), the chief difference between the two branches is that the Southern Branch continued to embrace sexual techniques (fang zhong) as the means of achieving longevity and immortality, while followers of the Northern Branch abjured their use. Zhang speculates that the change in practices of the Northern Branch may have occurred because, while Northern China was ruled by the Jin dynasty (A.D. 1115–1234), the King of Jin, who belonged to a minority nationality, suppressed the Taoist sexual practice. In addition to political pressure, there may have been economic pressure. At that time, Northern China was poorer than Southern China under the rule of the Southern Sung dynasty. Thus it may have been prohibitively expensive to buy the virgin girls and boys required for fully practicing fang zhong.

The major Taoist schools comprised numerous smaller sects; Fu (1975) lists 86 sects. Professor Zhou Shaoxian, who devoted decades to reading the entire *Taoist Canon*, comprising more than 1,600 books totaling 200,000 pages, mentions only two sects that used fang zhong. Both belonged to the Southern Branch of the Northern ("Perfect Realization") School (Zhou, 1982). Zhang Sanfeng and Zhao Liangpi (Ziyang Daoren) are the founders of these two sects, and the authors of *Zhang Sanfeng's Instructions in Physiological Alchemy* (San Feng Tan Chueh) and *Mental Images of the Mysteries and Subtleties of Sexual Techniques* (Hsuan Wei Hshin In), respectively. (The founder of the Taoist sect should not be confused with another man named Zhang Sanfeng, a famous master of marital arts who lived in the Sung dynasty.)

MYTHS—SOURCES OF TAOIST SEXUAL THEORY

Physicians and Other Experts

No later than the Han dynasty (206 B.C.–A.D. 220), and perhaps earlier, "fang-shu" was originated by "fang-shih" (alchemists and/or prescriptionists), "fang-zhong-jia" (experts on sexual techniques, or ancient sexologists), and medical doctors. It was then seen primarily as a medical art (Zhou Shaoxian, 1982; Hsu Ti-shan, 1977; Fu, 1975). As mentioned earlier, in Chapter 3, Pan Ku (A.D. 32–92), in *The History of the Former Han Dynasty,* included "fang zhong" in a special category listed just after the category for medicine, and described eight books devoted to sexual techniques. The later *History of the Sui Dynasty* simply includes such texts under the heading of "medical books."

The *History of the Later Han Dynasty* (Hou Han Shu), a standard history, contains several biographies of fang-shih, of which some excerpts follow.

Kan Shih, Tung-Kuo Yen-nien, and Feng Chun-ta

Kan Shih, Tung-Kuo Yen-nien, and Feng Chun-ta were all fang-shih. They were practitioners of Master Jung-cheng's arts of sexual regimen; they sometimes drank urine and sometimes suspended themselves upside down. They coveted every drop of seminal energy and were cautious neither to overexert their vision nor speak with exaggeration. Kan Shih, Yuan-fang [Tso Tz'u], and Yen-nien...all... lived from one to two hundred years of age. (Translated by De-Woskin, 1983)

Leng Shou Kuang

Leng was an outstanding practitioner of the arts of Jung Cheng.... The essential point of this art is to guard the life force and to nourish the chi by (relying on) the "Valley Spirit that never dies." When this is done white hairs become black again, and teeth that have dropped out are replaced by new ones. The art of commerce with women is to close the hands tightly and to refrain from ejaculation, causing the sperm to return and nourish the brain. (Translated by Needham, 1983)

Other pioneers of fang shu were such noted physicians as the above-mentioned Ge Hong, Tao Hongjing, and Sun Simiao.

Written Sources of Taoist Sexual Technique

Taoist sexual technical books can be divided into two categories. The first, listed in Table 4–1, consists of early Taoist resources written during the Han and Tang dynasties (206 B.C.–A.D. 907). These works were discussed in the previous chapter. The second, listed in Table 4–2, consists of Taoist sexual works that were written by the Taoist masters who were founders or major leaders of those sects which stressed a sexual regimen.

Tables 4–1 and 4–2 list extant Taoist sexual books in alphabetical order by title. All are listed in the References section of this book under the names of their authors and/or editors, which are given here in brackets.

The following discussion of Taoist sexual lore relies on these primary sources, using many direct quotations to accurately reproduce the content and flavor of these writings. The discussion is necessarily an introduction to the field. Most of the fang zhong texts are rare and thus not readily available, even in China. A detailed study of all these works, their background, and their impact on Chinese society would require a separate book. Most of the translations of the quotations are based on Ishihara and Levy (1968), van Gulik (1961), or Needham (1956, 1983), with some adaptations by the author. Translations by other authors are cited accordingly.

Table 4–1. Early Taoist Works on Sexual Technique

 1. Bao-pu-zi (Pao Po Tzu, Pao Phu Tzu, or Pao-p'u-tzu) (*The Work of Ko Hung, or Book of the Preservation-of-Solidarity Master*) [Ge Hong, 1965; Ware (Tr.), 1966.]

 2. Bei Ji Qian Jin Yao Fang (*Prescriptions Worth a Thousand Pieces of Gold for Emergencies*) Volume 27 Section 8: "Fang-nei-pu-i" ("The Benefits in the Bedchamber") [Sun Simiao, 1982.]

 3. Chou-i-ts'an-t'ung-chi (*Textual Research on the Taoistic and Magical Interpretation of the Book of Changes, or The Accordance of the Book of Changes with the Phenomena of Composite Things*) [Lu Guangrong, Lou Yugang, & Wu Jiachun (Eds.), 1987.]

 4. He-yin-yang-fang (*Methods of Intercourse between Yin and Yang*) [Zhou Yimiu, 1989.]

 5. Shi-wan (*Ten Questions and Answers*) [Zhou Yimiu, 1989.]

 6. Su Nu Ching (*Immaculate Girl Canon*) [Yeh Te-hui. (Ed.). 1914.]

 7. Su Nu Fang (*Immaculate Girl Prescriptions*) [Yeh Te-hui (Ed.), 1914.]

 8. Tian-xia-zhi-tao-tan (*Lectures on the Super Tao in the Universe*) [Zhou Yimiu, 1989.]

 9. Tung Hsuan Tzu (*Book of the Mystery-Penetrating Master*) [Yeh Te-hui (Ed.), 1914.]

 10. Yang Hsing Yen Ming Lu (*On Delaying Destiny by Nourishing the Natural Forces*) [Li Shihua & Shen Dehui (Eds.), 1987.]

 11. Yu Fang Chih Yao (*Important Matters of the Jade Chamber*) [Yeh Te-hui (Ed.), 1914.]

 12. Yu Fang Pi Chueh (*Secret Instructions Concerning the Jade Chamber*) [Yeh Te-hui (Ed.), 1914.]

METHODS—TAOIST SEXUAL LORE

In recent years, Western fascination with all things Oriental has included a curiosity about Taoist metaphysics. The martial arts, t'ai chi and chi kung, Chinese herbal medicine, and acupuncture have all gained wide acceptance. Those who explore sexual lore in the expectation of enhancing their own pleasure are sometimes drawn by the possibility that these techniques will indeed lengthen their lives. Suffice it to say that the Chinese belief that distant ancestors were exceptionally long-lived parallels similar myths of the ancient Greeks and Hebrews. A study of China's most ancient human fossils, the bones of Peking man, found that, of 40 individuals, the oldest had lived to be about 60 years old, a third had died by age 14, and a quarter had died between the ages of 30 and 50 (K. C. Chang, 1977; Ruan, 1977). While special mention will be made of sexual techniques that have practical value, we certainly are not advocating the use of Taoist prescriptions for immortality!

Each aspect of sexual lore is related to all the others. Each is conceived as one element of a total system, and all share elements derived from the underlying concepts of Yin-Yang and chi. For descriptive purposes, the entire system may be divided into eight categories of belief: (1) the myth that longevity and/or immortality are attainable by sexual activity; (2) the corollary myth that intercourse with virgins, preferably

Table 4–2. Works of the Later Taoist Masters

1. Chi Chi Chen Ching (*True Manual of the "Perfected Equalization"*) [Lu Dongbin, 1598.]
2. Fang Chung Lien Chi Chieh Yao (*Concise Instructions of Strengthening Oneself in the Bedchamber*) [Huayangzi (Ed.), 1936.]
3. Fang Shu Hsuan Chi (*The Mysterious Essence of Bedchamber Techniques*) [Huayangzi (Ed.), 1936.]
4. Hsiu Chen Yen I (*A Popular Exposition of the Methods of Regenerating the Primary Vitalities*) [Deng Xixian, 1598.]
5. Hsuan Wei Hshin In (*Mental Images of the Mysteries and Subtleties of Sexual Techniques*) [Zhao Liangpi (before 1850).]
6. Lu Tsu Wu Phien (*The Taoist Patriarch Lu Dongbin's Five Poetical Essays on Sexual Techniques*) [Lu Dongbin (before 1850).]
7. San Feng Tan Chueh (*Zhang Sanfeng's Instructions in the Physiological Alchemy*) [Zhang Sanfeng (before 1850).]
8. She Sheng Pi Phou (*Secret Instructions for Regimen*) [Huayangzi (Ed.), 1936.]
9. Wu Chen Pien (*Understanding Reality: A Taoist Alchemical Classic, or Poetical Essay on Realising the Necessity of Regenerating the Primary Vitalities*) [Zhang Baiduan, 1987; Cleary, 1987.]

young virgins, contributes to men's health; (3) the corollary belief in the desirability of multiple sexual partners; (4) the notions of "cai Yin pu Yang" (gathering a woman's Yin to nourish a man's Yang) and "cai Yang pu Yin" (gathering a man's Yang to nourish a woman's Yin); (5) the notion of the preciousness of "ching," or "seminal essence"; (6) the corollary belief in the possibility of "huan jing pu lau" (making the seminal essence return to nourish the brain); (7) the corollary belief in the value of preventing and interrupting ejaculation by pressing the "point" (in the perineal area); and (8) the belief that immense sexual satisfaction may be derived from coitus without ejaculation.

Many of the following passages become more meaningful when it is known that, in Taoist sexual books, the woman in her role as sexual partner was called "ding." The "ding" was originally a cooking vessel with two loop handles and three or four legs, which Taoist alchemists used as a reaction vessel. The use of the word in a discussion of longevity or immortality always refers to the female sex partner, and is one of many instances of parallel use of alchemical and sexual language.

Longevity and Immortality through Sexual Activity

Regarding the essential value of recommended methods of intercourse, the *Canon of the Immaculate Girl* says:

The King sent the Woman Selective to ask P'eng the Methuselah about the ways of prolonging life and benefiting old age. Said P'eng, "One achieves longevity by loving the essence, cultivating the spiritual, and partaking of many kinds of medicines. If you don't know the ways of intercourse, taking herbs is of no benefit. The producing of man and woman is like the begetting of Heaven and Earth. Heaven and Earth have attained the methods of intercourse and, therefore, they lack the limitation of finality. Man loses the method of intercourse and therefore suffers the mortification of early death. If you can avoid mortification and injury and attain the arts of sex, you will have found the way of nondeath."

In "The Ultimate System," the fifth chapter of *The Work of Ko Hung* (see Chapter 3), Ge Hong wrote in a similar vein:

A prime minister under the Han, Chang Tsang, happening to learn a minor recipe, lived to 180 by sucking his wives' milk.... Even if medicines are not obtainable and only breath circulation is practiced, a few hundred years will be attained provided the scheme is carried out fully, but one must also know the art of sexual intercourse to achieve such extra years. If ignorance of the sexual art causes frequent losses of sperm to occur, it will be difficult to have sufficient energy to circulate the breaths. (Ware, 1966)

In *Mental Images of the Mysteries and Subtleties of Sexual Techniques*, Zhao Lianpi (before 1850) asserted that the life span attainable through Taoist techniques is thousands of years long.

The Value of Virgins as Sex Partners

Almost all Taoist sex handbooks recommended that the "ding" should be a girl of 14 to 16, just before or after menarche. In *Zhang Sanfeng's Instructions in Physiological Alchemy*, "ding" were classified into three ranks. The lowest rank comprised women between the ages of 21 and 25. The middle rank comprised 16- to 20-year-old virgins after menarche. The highest rank comprised 14-year-old virgins before menarche.

Possibly numerology, as well as physiological maturity, was a factor in determining the ideal age of the female companion. In a poem in Mental Images, it was said that the first sexual partner should be 5,048 days old (i.e., just under 14). This book was most stringent in its requirements for a youthful "ding." The prose text stated that the ideal "ding" would be a girl who was 5,048 days old and had not reached menarche, and that no woman older than 18 was a suitable partner for sexual alchemy.

Westerners might think that these recommendations betrayed a rather obvious partiality to youthful beauty, but this was not the case. In fact, *Prescriptions* explicitly stated that youth and virginity are more valuable than attractiveness:

> The females with whom you will have intercourse do not need to be beautiful, but they must be adolescents who have undeveloped breasts and are well covered with flesh. They will prove advantageous.

In fact, intercourse with virgins, especially young virgins, was held to be beneficial because it was thought that their supply of Yin energy had not yet been depleted. That is the basis of the following recommendations in *Secret Instructions Concerning the Jade Chamber.*

> Now men who wish to obtain great benefits do well in obtaining women who don't know the Way. They also should initiate virgins (into sex), and their facial color will come to be like (the facial color of) virgins. However, (man) is only distressed by (a woman) who is not young. If he gets one above 14 or 15 but below 18 or 19, it is most beneficial. However, the highest (number of years) must not exceed 30. Those who, though not yet 30, have already given birth, cannot be beneficial (to the man). The masters preceding me, who transmitted the Way to each other, lived to be 3,000 years old. Those who combine this (method) with (use of) medicines can become immortal.

The Desirability of Multiple Female Partners

A number of texts cite the supposed longevity of culture heroes as proof of the value of multiple sex partners. Thus, for example, *Important Matters of the Jade Chamber* asserts that "Peng the Methuselah said, 'The Yellow Emperor had sex with twelve hundred women and ascended as an Immortal.' " But recall that Ge Hong, in *The Work of Ko Hung,* argued that this was not the sole cause of the Emperor's immortality, as the Emperor had also engaged in alchemy. (Ge Hong's skepticism is interesting in view of the fact that the very existence of the Yellow Emperor is a myth.)

The prescriptions for multiple partners were usually accompanied by reference to the idea that semen must be retained. Thus, for example, the Taoist Liu Ching was quoted in *Important Matters of the Jade Chamber* as saying, "Those, however, who do not emit in intercourse and in a day and a night have relations with several tens (of women) without losing their semen, completely cure all ailments and daily are benefited in longevity."

The reason for changing sex partners was the same as the reason for choosing young women and virgins—to assure a constant supply of Yin energy. So, for example, *Secret Instructions Concerning the Jade Chamber* said:

> The Green Ox Taoist said: "If you change women often, many are the benefits. It is especially beneficial if you have more than ten partners a night. If you constantly control the same woman, her emission force changes to a weak one, which cannot greatly benefit the man. It also causes the woman to become emaciated."

Prescriptions elaborated this point, explaining, "If a man continually has intercourse with one and the same woman, her Yin essence will become weak and she will be of little advantage to the man." The text goes on to point out the danger that the man's Yang will be overwhelmed by the woman's Yin.

> Yang is modeled after fire, Yin after water. Just as water can quench fire, so Yin can diminish Yang. If the contact lasts too long, the Yin essence (absorbed by the man) will grow stronger than his own Yang essence, whereby the latter will be harmed. Thus what the man loses through the sexual act will not be compensated by what he gains. If one can copulate with twelve women without once emitting semen, one will remain young and handsome forever. If a man can copulate with 93 women and still control himself, he will attain immortality.

Gathering Yin to Nourish Yang, and Yang to Nourish Yin

Most descriptions of Taoist sexual techniques are man-centered, referring only to "gathering woman's Yin to nourish man's Yang." Therefore, the emphasis, as just described, was on coitus with several partners in succession, culminating in a single ejaculation. Part of the rationale for prolonged intercourse was the notion that the woman's orgasm (khuai) strengthened the man's vital powers; just as the man "shed Yang" in orgasm, the woman "shed Yin." Hence the male act was to be prolonged as much as possible so that the Yang might be nourished by as much Yin as possible.

In the Taoist sex manuals, sexual intercourse was frequently described as a "battle." The ideal was for a man to "defeat" the "enemy" in the sexual "battle" by keeping himself under complete control so as not to emit semen, while at the same time exciting the woman till she reached orgasm and shed her Yin essence, which was then absorbed by the man. This approach is exemplified in the *True Manual of the "Perfected Equalization"*:

> "Throws the entire force into the battle" means that the woman's passion reaches its apex. Then the woman will shed her "true essence" completely and it is absorbed by me. In this case "chi chi" means that I have obtained the "true Yang." One "ji" means twelve years, every time a man obtains the "true Yang" during coitus his span of life will be prolonged by twelve years. The storeroom is the marrow, the height of strength is the ni-huan point in the brain. "Withdraw from the battlefield" means "descending from the horse." Thereafter the man should lie on his back and regulate his breath, moving his midriff so that the newly acquired vital essence flows up to the ni-huan and so strengthens his supply of life power. In this way he shall remain free from disease and attain longevity.

A Popular Exposition of the Methods of Regenerating the Primary Vitalities utilizes a different metaphoric language to describe the mystical benefits of loveplay in great detail:

> The Great Medicine of the Three Peaks: The upper is called the Red Lotus Peak, its medicine is named Jade Fountain, Jade Fluid, or Fountain of Sweet Spirits. This medicine emanates from the two cavities under a woman's tongue. Its color is gray....The man should swallow it....It will moisten his five viscera,...generating vital essence and new blood.
>
> The middle peak is called the Double Water Chestnut Peak and its medicine is called Peach of Immortality, White Snow, or also Coral Juice. This medicine emanates from the two breasts of a woman. Its color is white, its taste sweet and agreeable. Of the three peaks, this one should receive attention first. A woman who has not yet borne a child...will give the most benefit.
>
> The lower is called Peak of the Purple Agaric, also the Grotto of the White Tiger, or the Mysterious Gateway. Its medicine is called Black Lead, or Moon Flower. It is in the vagina. Usually it does not flow out. Only in coitus is it secreted. It is very good for the "Original Yang" and Spirit.
>
> This is the Great Medicine of the Three Peaks. Only the man who can control his passion and sexual excitement in coitus can obtain this medicine and achieve longevity.

There are some texts which detail how a woman may turn intercourse to her own benefit. Chapter 5 includes a description of a novel, *Unofficial History of the Bamboo Garden,* whose plot hinges on a woman's exploitation of her sexual partners. A Taoist text describing the technique by which a woman may gather men's Yang is *Secret Instructions Con-*

cerning the Jade Chamber, which attributes these remarks to "Harmony Master Chung":

> Not only should the male element be nourished, but the female element should likewise be. The Queen Mother of the West nourished the female element and used the method. Once she had intercourse with a male, the male immediately became ill, but her facial color became shiny and glossy.
>
> The Queen Mother of the West had no husband, and she liked to have intercourse with virgin youths. Therefore, even though it's not a part of the world's teachings, how could it have been (known to) the Queen Mother alone? (i.e., although the method may not have been commonly known, it is unlikely that the queen alone knew this technique. Anyone could accomplish what she did by following the correct Way.)
>
> In having intercourse with a man, (the woman) should tranquilize her heart and settle her intent. If, for example, the male is not yet excited, you must wait till he becomes agitated. Therefore, control your feelings somewhat so as to respond in concert with him. In any event, you must not shake and dance about, causing your female fluid to be exhausted first.

There is a rare passage in Yun-chi-chi-chien (*The Seven Bamboo Tablets of the Cloudy Satchel,* an important collection of Taoist material edited by Chang Chun-fang in A.D. 1020), quoted by van Gulik (1961), which describes the process of gathering the opposite essence as completely identical for both the man and the woman, rather than limiting the woman to the passive role of having her Yin essence stirred and activated by the man:

> After they have concentrated and purified their thoughts, then a man and a woman may practise together the art that leads to longevity. This method... allows a man and a woman together to activate their chi and the man to nurture his semen (ching) and the woman her 'blood'.... The two partners should begin by meditating, detaching their mind from their own body and all worldly things. Then they grind their teeth seven times and recite the following spell: "May the Golden Essence of the White Origin bring my Five Flowers to life; may the Yellow Lord of the Centre harmonize my soul and regulate my essence; may the Supreme Essence of the Great Emperor solidify my humours and fortify my spirit; may the Unsurpassed Supreme True One bind my six chi; may the Mysterious Old Man of the Supreme Essence make the spirit return and thus strengthen the brain. Make the two of us unite and blend so that the embryo is refined and the Treasure conserved." Having pronounced this spell, the man holds his reins and locks his semen, so that the translated chi ascends along the spinal column till it reaches the ni-huan spot

in the brain. This is called "making it return to the Origin" (huan-yuan). The woman controls her emotions and nurtures her spirit so that she does not reach the climax ("the refined fire does not move"); she makes the chi of her two breasts descend into her reins, then again ascend from there till it has reached her ni-huan point. This is called "transforming the true" (hua-chen). The elixir (tan) thus formed (in the bodies of the two participants) if nurtured for a hundred days, will become transcendental (ling). And if this discipline is continued over a very long period, then it will become a natural habit, the method for living long and attaining Immortality.

The Preciousness of "Ching" (Seminal Essence)

One of the goals of Taoist sexual techniques was to increase the amount of "life-giving" ching as much as possible by sexual stimulation, simultaneously avoiding its loss. While some foregoing passages discussed the importance of retaining ching in connection to the practice of intercourse with multiple partners, the technique of retention was important in itself.

Secret Instructions Concerning the Jade Chamber described the pleasures of orgasm as temporary and ultimately debilitating, in contrast to the benefits of seminal retention:

> The Woman Selective said, "In intercourse, semen emission is regarded as pleasurable. Now if one closes it off and doesn't emit, what kind of pleasure can there be?"
>
> Replied P'eng the Methuselah: "When semen is emitted, the body is fatigued, the ears are pained and deafened with noise, and the eyes are pained and on the verge of sleep. The throat is completely dry and the joints are slackened. Though one is restored, it is but for a short while, and the joy ends in dissatisfaction. Now if one moves but doesn't emit, life force and vigor are in excess, the body is well accommodated, and the ears and eyes are sharpened. While stressing quietude, you can again establish what you love in your heart. Since it is always insufficient (to quell your desire through emission), how can this (non-emission) be other than pleasurable?"

In the same book, the Woman Plain tells the Yellow Emperor that the benefits increase with each intercourse that takes place without ejaculation:

> "If you move but don't emit, then your life force and vigor are strengthened. If again you move but don't emit, your ears and eyes are sharpened. If a third time...all sicknesses vanish. If a fourth time... the five internal organs [the liver, heart, spleen, lungs, and kidneys]

are all pacified. An eighth time..., the body begins to glow. If a ninth
time..., longevity will not be lost. If a tenth time you move but don't
emit, you can communicate with the gods.

In accord with this line of reasoning, *Prescriptions* describes seminal
retention as simple prudence, remarking:

> But if a man does not control himself and emits semen every
> time he sleeps with a woman, it is as if he were taking away oil from
> a lamp already nearly burnt out....Young men do not know this
> rule and those who know it do not practise it. Then, when they have
> reached middle age and when they have come to understand this
> principle, it is already too late.

The Value of Making Seminal Essence "Return to the Brain"

The method of seminal retention was an interesting one, which has
been used in other cultures as a contraceptive technique. At the moment
of ejaculation, pressure was exerted on the urethra in the perineal area,
thus diverting the seminal secretion into the bladder. The Taoists thought
that the seminal essence could thus be made to ascend and revivify the
upper parts of the body: that is why the practice was termed "huan jing
pu nao"—making the jing return to restore the brain.

In *The Work of Ko Hung*, Ge Hong described this method as essential,
remarking:

> On the technology of sex at least ten authors have written, some
> explaining how it can replenish and restore injuries and losses, others
> telling how to cure many diseases by its aid, others again describing
> the gathering of the Yin force to benefit the Yang, others showing
> how it can increase one's years and protract one's longevity. But the
> great essential here is making the semen return to nourish the brain
> (huan ching pu nao), a method which the adepts have handed down
> from mouth to mouth, never committing it to writing. If a man does
> not understand this art he may take the most famous [macrobiotic]
> medicines, but he will never achieve longevity or immortality.

An extremely detailed description of the method is found in *Important Matters of the Jade Chamber:*

> Xian Jing (*The Manuals of the Immortals*) describe the way of mak-
> ing the ching return to nourish the brain. During sexual intercourse,
> when the jing (semen) has become very agitated and is on the point
> of coming out, strong pressure must be applied with the two middle
> fingers of the left hand to a spot behind the scrotum and in front of
> the anus, while at the same time the breath should be fully expelled

through the mouth, none being retained (in the lungs), and the teeth gnashed several dozen times. Thus the ching will be emitted, but not to the outside world, for it will come back from the Stalk of Jade and mount upwards to enter the brain.

Pressing the Point

As can be seen in the foregoing quotation, the technique of "pressing the point" was valued because it aided in the goal of seminal retention. There were numerous variations on this technique; the following is quoted from *Prescriptions:*

> Every time a man feels that he is about to emit semen during the sexual act, he should close his mouth and open his eyes wide, hold his breath, and firmly control himself. He should move both hands up and down and hold his breath in his nose, constraining the lower part of his body so that he breathes with his abdomen. Straightening his spine he should quickly press the Ping-i Point [located about one inch above the nipple of the right breast] with index and middle finger of his left hand, then let out his breath, at the same time gnashing his teeth a thousand times.

Sexual Satisfaction from Coitus without Ejaculation

The authors of the texts recommending coitus without ejaculation clearly felt the need to answer the question they frequently ascribed to participants in their dialogues—"How can this type of intercourse give pleasure?" They answered with detailed descriptions of techniques which, while delaying orgasm, would contribute to the pleasure of the participants. They often emphasized slow, gentle movements. For example, *Important Matters of the Jade Chamber* contains the following passage:

> The Taoist Liu Ching said, "In general, the way to control women is first to strive to play and amuse gently, causing the spiritual (qualities) to harmonize and the intent to feel moved. After a good long while (of this), you can have intercourse and insert the jade stalk within. Strong and firm, suddenly withdrawing; make your entries and withdrawals relaxed and slow. Do not expel your semen (like dashing something down) from the heights."

Because the woman's orgasm was important, passages like the following excerpt from the *Book of the Mystery-Penetrating Master* also detailed the manner in which the man could adapt his actions to the woman's level of excitement:

...The man prostrates himself on top of her and kneels inside her thighs....The man then rapidly inserts and quickly pierces; he thrusts in and out, elevating his waist. He awaits the woman's agitation and adapts the slowness and quickness (of his movements) accordingly....the woman's emission fluid should overflow. The male should then withdraw; he cannot revert to death [allow the penis to become flaccid after ejaculation] but must return to life [avoid ejaculation and retain an erection]. A deathlike emission is largely injurious to the male. One should be especially cautious (to remove the penis from within the vagina while it is still hard). (Author's translation)

TAOIST TECHNIQUES FOR SEXUAL PLEASURE

The Taoist techniques for stimulating pleasure were conditioned by the belief that "the way of nourishing the life is by means of the Yin and the Yang" ("Ying Yang yang seng chih tao"). This meant that the two great forces Yin and Yang, as incarnated in individual humans, each provided indispensable nourishment for the other. As just explained, the practice of the principle meant that it was equally desirable for a woman to have orgasms, and for her male partner to be sexually stimulated while delaying ejaculation as long as possible. Though they obviously failed to achieve their larger goals, the Taoist adepts really did succeed in their ancillary aims of developing techniques for delaying male orgasm and sexually arousing women. Some of the skills are described in the remainder of this chapter.

Mastering the Differences in Male and Female Sexual Response

A crucial point made in the Taoist texts was that it is important to understand the differences between male and female sexual responses and capacities. The *Canon of the Immaculate Girl* said:

The reason for the decline of men is only that they all abuse the ways of female-male element intercourse. Now woman's superiority to man (in this respect) is like water's extinguishing fire. If you understand this and carry it out, you will be like the cauldrons and the tripods, which harmonize well the five flavors and thereby achieve a broth of meat and vegetables.

Seductiveness and sensitivity to individual moods were also stressed, as in the following passage from *A Popular Exposition of the Methods of Regenerating the Primary Vitalities:*

> The feelings of woman lie deeply hidden. How can one rouse them and how can one know when they have been roused? In order to rouse them one should follow the method of first serving a light liqueur to someone who desires strong wine. Affectionate women should be made even more tender by sweet discourses, greedy women should be excited by costly presents. Woman's feelings are naturally ruled by no fixed principle, they are always easily influenced by what they see.

"Harmonizing the Will"

The ideal emotional atmosphere of intercourse itself was one of relaxed cooperation in a mutuality known as "harmonizing the will," that is, the respective desires of the two partners. The *Canon of the Immaculate Girl* described the ideal intercourse in the following manner:

> If you wish to know its ways, they are in settling the life force, tranquilizing the mind, and harmonizing the will. If the three phenomena are all attained, your spirit is unified; neither cold or hot, hungry or satiated, your body is regulated and fixed, and sex is always leisurely and relaxed. Shallow insertions and leisurely movements, and few ins and outs; the woman has pleasurable feelings, and the man flourishes and doesn't deteriorate. Through this they attain their climax.
>
> ...The female and male elements respond only through being moved reciprocally. Therefore, if the female element can't be secured, the male element is displeased; if the male element can't be secured, the female element doesn't get excited. If the man wishes intercourse but the woman is displeased, or if the woman wishes intercourse but the man does not, their two hearts are not in harmony and they are not moved to emit. Furthermore, if you go up unexpectedly or go down suddenly (in emotion), the pleasures of love are not given. If the man wishes to seek the woman and the woman wishes to seek the man, their feelings and intent combine as one, and together they achieve delight at heart.

Combining Male Relaxation and Female Excitement

The sexual adepts freely admitted that it was a difficult challenge for a man to maintain self-control while exciting his partner's passion.

They detailed physical and mental techniques for solving the problem. For example, the *True Manual of the "Perfected Equalization"* said:

> In the Taoist master's sexual "battle" (to give the woman an orgasm while avoiding ejaculation), his enemy is the woman. He should begin by touching her vulva, kissing her lips and tongue, and touching her breasts, making her highly aroused. But he should keep himself under control, his mind as detached as if it were floating in the azure sky, his body sunk into nothingness. He must close his eyes, avoid looking at the woman, and maintain an utter nonchalance so that his own passion is not roused.
>
> When she makes sexual movements, the man must remain still rather than take any action. When her hand actively touches the penis, the man avoids her caress. The man can employ stillness and relaxation, to overcome the woman's excitement and movement.

A Popular Exposition of the Methods of Regenerating the Primary Vitalities was even more extreme in its recommendations, construing any emotional attachment as a mere impediment to the metaphysical goals of intercourse:

> When a man first begins to engage in sexual intercourse he must use every means to suppress all lustful thoughts. He must choose as his partner a woman who is ugly so that she does not excite his passion and does not give him intense pleasure. In that way the man will easily learn how to control himself.
>
> Every man who has obtained a beautiful "crucible" will naturally love her with all his heart. But every time he copulates with her he should force himself to think of her as ugly and hateful. (Author's translation)

Studying the Woman's Sexual Responses to Choose the Perfect Moment for Penetration

Just as stimulation of the woman was a calculated attempt to maximize the amount of Yin available to the man, knowledge of her response was taken as a means for choosing an auspicious moment to gather her Yin. *Instructions Concerning the Jade Chamber* describes the signs of physiological arousal, and the manner of penetration, in considerable detail:

> The ways of sexual intercourse are not especially strange. But you should be composed and at tranquil ease, esteeming harmoniousness. You play with the pubic region, try to kiss her deeply, and thrust forward with the tongue and lightly glide with it in order to excite her. When a woman is moved by a man, there is evidence. Her ears get as hot as if she has drunk a strong wine; her breasts

rise in warmth, and if you grasp them they fill your hands. The nape
of her neck frequently moves, her legs are wildly brandished about,
her licentious overflow appeals, and she presses on the man's body.
At a time like this, if you draw back slightly and are shallow (in
penetration), the penis gains the life force and the female element is
disadvantaged.

Appropriate Positions and Movements

A variety of positions and movements for intercourse were all described in accordance with the principles just outlined.

For example, *True Manual of the "Perfected Equalization"* gives concrete descriptions as follows:

> When she becomes very aroused and excited and her desire for
> the penis is strong, he changes his posture, lies on his back, and lets
> her take the woman-superior position and move actively. He keeps
> still, closing his eyes and mouth.
>
> Closing (his) eyes and mouth, withdrawing (his) hands and feet,
> pressing the seminal duct between (his) fingers while concentrating
> (his) mind, he is like a turtle withdrawing into itself. As to the serpent
> swallowing its prey, it will first suck and nibble at its victim till it is
> completely powerless, then swallow it never to let it go again. When
> a tiger is about to grab its prey, it fears that the victim will detect
> him. Therefore the tiger crouches in concealment and silently lies in
> wait. In that manner its prey will never escape.
>
> When she is almost ready to climax, he returns to the man-
> superior position. Then, when she has had her orgasm, without ejacu-
> lation he repeats the battle again and again until she is too exhausted
> to continue.

Controlled Breathing

In such sexual handbooks as *The Mysterious Essence of Bedchamber
Techniques* and *Secret Instructions of Sexual Regimen,* there appear five Chinese characters, each describing a mode of breathing, each a key part of
the effort to delay male ejaculation. Each of these characters has multiple
translations, given in parentheses: "cun" (keep, remain, and reserve), "suo"
(draw back, withdraw, and recoil), "chou" (take out, or obtain by draw-
ing), "xi" (breathe in, draw, and suck up), and "bi" (close, stop up).

"Cun" is a type of slow breathing; "suo" involves inhaling through
the nose and holding the breath; during "xi" one uses his penis to

absorb Yin substance; and in "bi" refrains from breathing through the mouth during the action of intercourse. (Author's translation)

The use of these techniques required considerable practice and discipline. According to *Mental Images of the Mysteries and Subtleties of Sexual Techniques:*

> Before one is ready to have sex with a partner, he must practice Taoist physiological alchemy. He must train his breathing for a hundred days. His breathing should become as smooth and well-balanced as possible. (Author's translation)

CONCLUSION—MODERN USES OF TAOIST SEXUAL METHODS

While some of the sexual information described in the Taoist handbooks is not correct, the major practical suggestions are definitely useful. Use of several of these techniques can prolong the sexual act and contribute to the pleasure of both partners. That is why many modern sex therapists use Taoist sexual teachings as a way to treat premature ejaculation and other sexual dysfunctions.

The Taoist texts may serve another purpose when they are finally made available to the Chinese people. Because they represent a historic heritage, they may be even more welcome than Western sex manuals. As we shall see in a later chapter, there is currently much sexual dissatisfaction as a direct result of enforced ignorance. Not only is the average length of intercourse short, but often there is little foreplay. The techniques which Taoists used in coldly calculated fashion may some day be learned and used in a sincere effort for mutual satisfaction.

Chapter 5

Prostitution in Chinese Society
From Acceptance to Persecution

THE ORIGINS AND DEVELOPMENT OF PROSTITUTION IN CHINA

References to prostitution in the ancient histories are so brief and vague that it is difficult to determine when and how the practice originated, but it is possible to speculate about the development of government-owned brothels. Some researchers believe that China's first brothels were established in the seventh century B.C. by the famous statesman and philosopher Guan Zhong (?–645 B.C.), who used them as a means of increasing the state's income. Guan, who was the premier of the State of Chi in the period of Duke Huan (reigning 681–643 B.C.), established seven government-owned markets with housing for 700 women in Duke Huan's palace (Wang, 1934; Bullough & Bullough, 1987). However, it is possible that the women's markets in Duke Huan's palace were not public brothels, but proof of his sexual extravagance (van Gulik, 1961). Other scholars suggest that institutionalized prostitution in China began in the Western Han dynasty, when the famous Emperor Wu (reigning 140–87 B.C.) recruited female camp followers for his armies; these women were called "ying-chi" ("camp harlots") (Chen, 1928; van Gulik, 1961). Some would place the institution of camp followers still earlier, in the Warring States period, when the King of Yue established a widows camp on a mountain to supply sexual outlets for his armies, possibly setting the precedent for Emperor Wu's camp harlots (Chen, 1928; Wang, 1934).

However the custom started, it is clear that the institution of government-run prostitution reached its peak in the Tang and Sung dynasties. In the Tang dynasty, some prostitutes were connected with local governments, and their lives and business activities were almost totally controlled by local officials. Another class of prostitutes were controlled by the imperial government; they lived in Pingkangli, a special district of Changan (the capital), and had greater freedom to conduct their own business (Gao, 1987). Private, commercial prostitution became most highly developed during the Ming and Ching dynasties. In this later era, the cities of Suzhou, Hangzhou, Nanjing, Yangzhou, Shanghai, Beijing, Tianjin, and Kuangzhou were all famous for their flourishing trade in prostitution.

THE COURTESANS

In ancient China, where most women had no opportunity to acquire an education and formal contact between men and women was frowned upon, it was the role of the courtesan to entertain a man and be his friend. Every prominent official, writer, artist, or merchant customarily left his wife at home when he traveled; instead, he was accompanied by one or more women skilled in making men feel comfortable. Courtesans with literary, musical, or dancing ability were especially desirable companions, and many became famous historical figures. Some of the better-known courtesans are described in the following biographies:

Chao Fei-yan

Chao Fei-yan (Flying Swallow Chao) was working in a "Song and Dancing House" when the Emperor Han Cheng Ti (reigned 32–7 B.C.) first heard rumors of her beauty. When Cheng Ti visited her for the first time, he went disguised as the servant of one of his nobles, in order to avoid any possible scandal. When he first saw her, the emperor was so dazzled by Chao Fei-yan's charm and beauty that he was speechless. Within a few days, he had the nobleman bring her to the imperial palace, where she became one of the queen's ladies-in-waiting. That very night, Cheng Ti summoned Chao Fei-yan to his Royal Bedchamber. He was so fascinated by her beauty that for the first few hours he simply gazed at her. During their love-making, Fei-yan enchanted the emperor with her sexual technique; she made him feel that intercourse was effortless, yet utterly satisfying. Soon the emperor made Fei-yan one of his official consorts, and eventually he found her so indispensable that he demoted the original queen and put Fei-yan in her place. Fei-yan is notable in Chinese history as a prostitute who became a queen. (Chou, 1971; Wang & Zhou, 1983)

Hsueh Tao

Hsueh Tao, who lived from A.D. 768 to 831, was so accomplished that she was able to compose sophisticated poetry when she was only nine years old. Her father, an official, took her with him when he was sent to a post in Sichuan Province, where he died, leaving her destitute. She registered as a prostitute in Chengtu, the provincial capital, and soon became famous for her wit and beauty. Some of the greatest poets of the day visited Hsueh Tao when they were in Sichuan and she became the favourite of the great general Wei Kao (A.D. 745–805), who was military governor of the province for many years. She invented a new kind of ornamental paper, used for writing poetry, that still bears her name, and her poems continue to be published. (van Gulik, 1961)

Li Shih-shih

During the reign of Emperor Huei Tsung (A.D. 1101–1125) of the Sung dynasty, Li Shih-shih was known as the most attractive prostitute in the imperial capital of Kaifeng. At the age of eighteen or nineteen, she excelled in playing the Chinese lyre. "Delicate as an orchid and graceful as a peony," Li Shih-shih was able to captivate many a court official with a single smile or a few words. Those who were fortunate enough to sleep with her said that she was also a "delicate orchid" in bed. After having made love to Shih-shih, Prime Minister Li Pang-yen said, "You feel utterly helpless when you make love to her. Her skin is as smooth as silk all over, giving you delight the moment your body touches hers. She knows when to be gentle, when to be vigorous and when to let herself go." The emperor became so enamored of Shih-shih that he disregarded the advice of several ministers and the jealousy of his queen and concubines to make love with her at every opportunity. When one of his concubines asked him what was so different about Shih-shih, the emperor replied, "None of you knows about the art of love. With her, I never have to labour, and yet she offers me so much pleasure. In bed, she is always so lively and so full of fun. Compared with her, all of you are like beauties made of clay or wood." (Chou, 1971; Wang & Zhou, 1983)

THE PROSTITUTES

Despite the glowing descriptions of their sexual artistry, the courtesans' primary role was as companions who were entertaining in private and presentable in public. However, the prostitutes working in privately owned brothels mainly provided sexual services. From the Sung to the Ming dynasties, government-run and privately owned prostitution existed side by side in China. Early in the Ching dynasty, from A.D. 1651 to 1673, the Manchu Emperors Shun-chih and Kang-hsi gradually abolished both local and imperial governmental involvement in prostitution; thus, for most of the Ching dynasty, prostitution in China was a private enterprise (Wang, 1934). For most of the Republican period in mainland China (1912–1949), some prostitutes were registered and others plied their trade illegally.

It is difficult to estimate the actual number of prostitutes in ancient China at any one time. Marco Polo, the Italian who traveled to China in the thirteenth century, reported that in the capital city of Peking there were over 20,000 women earning a living through prostitution, and in Hangzhou there were so many he could not estimate their number. Though Polo's estimate may have been exaggerated, there is little doubt that prostitution played an important part in Chinese life during the ancient and medieval periods (Bullough & Bullough, 1987).

Some statistics on prostitution were compiled during the Republican era, and a sample of this information is presented in Tables 5–1, 5–2, and 5–3.

Table 5–1. Registered Public Prostitutes in Peking

Year	Brothels	Total number of prostitutes	First	Second	Third	Fourth
			Rank[a]			
1917	391	3,500[b]				
1918	406	3,880				
1929	332	3,752	328	528	1,895	301

[a]Those in the first rank were the most expensive "high-class" prostitutes; those in the fourth rank were the inexpensive streetwalkers.
[b]Underground prostitutes numbered about 7,000 in 1917.

Table 5–2. Registered Public Prostitutes in Shanghai in 1920

Total	First	Second	Third	Fourth
	Rank			
60,141	1,200	490	37,161	21,315

Table 5–3. Registered Public Prostitutes in Canton in 1926

Brothels	Number of prostitutes	First	Second	Third
		Rank		
131	1,362[a]	761	468	115

[a]Underground prostitutes numbered about 2,600.

SEXUAL PRACTICES OF CHINESE PROSTITUTES

Sexual Techniques Used by Chinese Prostitutes

One of the best descriptive summaries of the prostitutes' art was contained in *Memoirs of the Plum Blossom Cottage,* the work of a nineteenth-century scholar using the pseudonym "Master of Plum Blossoms." He used the character of a procuress to give this explicit account:

As most males want to deem themselves potent and virile, your primary concern is *not* to hurt their ego. Since they are your customers, your job is to satisfy their desires, not yours. Let them imagine they have the initiative, though in fact it is in your hands. With someone who does not have the stamina, you must feign satisfaction even though he may discharge the moment he enters you. You can still let his shrunken organ remain inside, embracing and caressing him as if he were the most wonderful man you had ever had. With a customer who has a tiny organ, you have to hold your legs tightly together once he puts it inside you. This will give him the feeling that his every thrust really hurts and yet thrills you. An older customer may find it difficult to keep an erection; in this case you will have to fondle his organ tenderly and gently. Meanwhile tell some sexy stories to give him time to warm up. If this fails to arouse him, you will have to use your mouth to suck it. If sucking still fails, you should gently advise him to sleep first and then have intercourse whenever he wakes up. Generally, a man is more potent after some rest. Never give him aphrodisiacs, for it will ruin his health. Besides, his inability is none of your responsibility, since you have tried all you can. But with a man who is really virile and has endurance, you have to rely on your techniques most. Do not let yourself be carried away even if he makes you enjoy it. For your own good, you have to make him discharge as quickly as you can. You must take the initiative without his knowledge. You can move your hips like a millstone in action, holding his waist tightly and stroking his spine near the waist gently but persistently. Meanwhile, you can tickle the roof of his mouth with the tip of your tongue. If you do all things skillfully, he will definitely discharge at your will. But be sure to let him have some fun, or his ego will be pricked and you will lose a customer. Some customers may arrive after having taken aphrodisiacs; therefore, you must not forget to make them drink a cup of white chrysanthemum tea before you take them to bed. Also remember that some wines can counter the effects of aphrodisiacs. With a man who has a big weapon, there is no cause for worry. This does not necessarily mean that he is extraordinarily virile. But for your own protection, slip behind the bed curtains and anoint your private parts with a sufficient amount of rose-petal ointment. Make sure that he knows nothing about this, for most customers like to show off the bigness of their weapons and enjoy whatever pain they may cause you. When you want to make him discharge quickly, just use the millstone tactics. You can slightly bend your waist so that his member will not reach too deep inside. When you are lucky enough to have a "spring chicken" (meaning virgin boy), you must be patient in coaching him. He is bound to be clumsy and may not be able to find the right path. Help him and make him overcome his initial shyness and lack of confidence. Sometimes, he can be more manly after his premature discharge. You must make him find both physical and mental pleasures in having sex. More often than not, you will find "spring chickens" most enjoyable after you have successfully coached them. (Translation adapted from Chou, 1971)

There are many descriptions of prostitutes who were said to have special sexual skills. For example, the well-known Shanghai prostitute Shilihong was known for her innocent schoolgirl beauty, and her exceptional control of her vaginal muscles. Shilihong could contract and relax her muscles in a manner that moved her customer's penis in and out without his moving; the sensation was said to be like sucking. Shilihong's customers needed to make appointments weeks in advance of seeing her. Another Shanghai prostitute, Zhang Fuzeng, was popular although she was already in her thirties and not particularly attractive. She was famous for her skill in oral sex; her customers said that she could roll her tongue into a hollow cylinder, then extend her lips more than an inch. She could make all sorts of movements, and make her customer's pleasure last quite a long time. Both men and women sought her services (Zhu, 1971).

The Training of Prostitutes

The female managers of some brothels had detailed manuals for the training of prostitutes. Zhonghua (1925) cited a manual used in the cities of Suzhou, Yangzhou, and Shanghai as an excellent example. The manual, based on the accumulated experiences of many prostitutes, asserted that a woman must meet the following basic requirements to be a successful prostitute:

1. SE (beauty): Natural beauty is rare. Focus on artificial beauty, especially on manner, posture, and expression;
2. YI (art, skill): Learn the methods of getting customers to stay with you for a long time;

3. QING (emotion, affection, passion): Be false about the truth, and true about falsehood (i.e., disguise one's true emotions, and express false sentiments with apparent sincerity), changeable, and lively;
4. BIANTAI (variation of attitudes): Be deceptive and heartless in dealings with customers. (Translated from Zhonghua, 1925, Vol. 3)

The manual goes on to describe every aspect of a prostitute's business in great detail, including instructions on how to walk, sit, and lie down gracefully, when to smile, how to sing, make conversation, apply cosmetics, and dress enticingly, how to conduct a flirtation, and how to manipulate customers.

The female procurers of Peking and Tientsin paid less attention to manners, emphasizing instead the acquisition of skill in sexual techniques. They used the *Canon of the Immaculate Girl* (Su Nu Jing) as a textbook, as well as live demonstrations to teach the prostitutes a variety of sexual positions, movements in coitus, and control of breathing (Zhonghua, 1925, Vol. 3).

Kang (1988a) reports her experience that brothel owners secretly gave their unwitting employees a medicine believed to cause sterility.

THE ABOLITION OF PROSTITUTION IN THE 1950s

When the Chinese Communists took power, one of the first social changes they introduced was the abolition of prostitution. Only one month after the Communist army took control of Beijing on February 3, 1949, the new municipal government announced a policy of limiting and controlling the brothels. On October 1, 1949, the founding of the People's Republic of China was declared, and less than eight weeks later, more than 2,000 Beijing policemen raided and closed all 224 of the city's brothels, arresting 1,286 prostitutes and 424 owners, procurers, and pimps (Beijing Public Security Bureau, 1988). Other cities soon followed suit. For example, in Shanghai, China's most populous city, there were 5,333 arrests of prostitutes between 1950 and 1955 (*Centre Daily News*, January 24, 1989).

The Communists believed that prostitution is caused by socioeconomic factors. Thus their initial policies emphasized eliminating the socioeconomic causes of prostitution by relieving the peasants of the debts, exorbitant rents, and other financial pressures that had forced them to sell their daughters into prostitution. The government gave former prostitutes free medical treatment for venereal disease. According to the Beijing Public Security Bureau (1988), a survey of 1,303 prostitutes in Beijing in 1950 found that 96.5% had nonspecific venereal infections, 84.9% had syphilis, and 53.8% had active gonorrhea. They were treated, usually with penicillin, by a special corps of 56 physicians and nurses who succeeded in curing 40% of the syphilis patients and 95% of the gonorrhea patients. Steps were taken to prevent those who had not been cured from spreading infection. Next, the women were given vocational training and new jobs. It was hoped that by using this method, the "New Society" could transform former prostitutes into "new persons." In the 1950s it was proclaimed that there were no prostitutes in the "New China," and in the early 1960s, Communist Party officials boasted that sexually transmitted diseases had disappeared from mainland China.

Although reforming prostitutes and eliminating sexually transmitted disease are laudable goals, the Communists were mistaken in describing prostitution as the rotten fruit of capitalism. If that is what it is, how can they explain the occurrence of prostitution in precapitalist societies and the recent reappearance of prostitution in "socialist" China? Clearly, the existence of prostitution does not depend on the prevalence of capitalism, socialism, or any other economic order. It is a phenomenon that can exist in many diverse societies—there is no need to put a political label on it.

In October 1957, in a new attempt to maintain order, the 81st Session of the Standing Committee of the First National People's Congress adopted a new law entitled Rules on the Control of and Punishment Concerning Public Security of the People's Republic of China (Cohen, 1968). The legislation announced the following policy on banning prostitution:

> Article 5: A person who commits any of the following acts disrupting public order shall be punished by detention of not more than ten days, a fine of not more than twenty yuan [Chinese currency unit] or a warning:...
> (8) Engaging in prostitution or having sexual relations with a woman secretly engaged in prostitution in violation of the government order repressing prostitution.

In 1979, at its Second Session, the Fifth National People's Congress adopted the first criminal law in Red China, The Criminal Law of the People's Republic of China, which took effect January 1, 1980 (Fang, 1982). Under this law, the punishment for prostitution is more severe:

> Chapter IV: Acts Against the Personal and Democratic Rights of Citizens
> Article 140: Whoever forces a female to engage in prostitution shall be sentenced to a fixed term of imprisonment of 3 to 10 years.

This law is little more than a piece of paper. At any time, the law's provisions can be changed by the political leadership; depending on their own feelings and opinions and their political needs, they may impose harsher punishments on pimps and owners of underground brothels, who are included in Article 140, or choose to punish prostitutes and their customers, who are not listed in the article at all (see the following).

THE REVIVAL OF PROSTITUTION IN THE 1980s

The severe repression of prostitution did not prevent its accelerated revival in the late 1970s and throughout the 1980s. The Public Security Department of the People's Republic of China ordered a nationwide police crackdown on prostitution in June 1981 and again in June 1982. The first official report of the recurrence and development of prostitution in mainland China appeared in March 1983. This document, which was written by the Public Security Department of the People's Republic of China and the National Association of Chinese Women, reported:

> According to the incomplete statistics from the three largest cities, Beijing, Shanghai, Tianjin, and four provinces, Kuangdong, Fujian, Zheijiang, and Liaoning, from January 1982 to November 1982, more than 11,500 persons were discovered to be involved in prostitution. More than 1,200 persons were owners and pimps of underground brothels; more than 4,200 women were prostitutes; and 1,800 persons, including 223 visitors from foreign countries and Hong Kong and Macao, were customers of prostitutes. There were 691 arrests, 662 sentences to labor camps, 790 detentions, and more than 1,500 fines. More than 900 underground brothels were banned and closed. An estimated 322 pornographic films and videotapes, and more than 100,000 assorted pornographic magazines, books, photos, and sex toys confiscated. According to surveys in the provinces of Kuangdong, Fujian, Zheijiang, and Hunan, more than half the cities and counties have already discovered prostitution. According to the survey of Jiangsu and Sichuan provinces, 50–60% of the prostitutes came from rural areas. In one village in Ho County, Guangxi Province, which has a total of 67 families, 35 women from 28 families had moved to cities to engage in prostitution. (Author's translation)

The author of this book is an eyewitness to the revival of prostitution in mainland China. As a pioneer sexologist and one of the leading experts in this field in China, he was the main speaker at the first national workshop on sex education, held in Shanghai in August 1985. There he was invited by the Shanghai Public Security Bureau to visit the Shanghai Women Delinquents Correctional Institution.

This Institution was founded in July 1984 and began receiving prisoners in September 1984. By the time the author visited in August 1985, the Institution had a staff of more than 30 and 150 inmates; it is antic-ipated that there will be a maximum of 40 staff members and 400 in-mates. Of the 150 women residing in the institution, about 100 were prostitutes, and the remaining 50 women were "sexual criminals" of var-ious kinds.

As the invited "temporary counselor," the author was asked by Mr. Li, the director of the Institution, to interview three women to investigate their frequent attacks on instructors in the Institution. One of these women, Ms. Za, was a sex "criminal" who will be intro-duced in Chapter 8. The other two, Ms. L. and Ms. Zu, were prosti-tutes. These two cases, while interesting and illustrative of the lives of prostitutes, are not necessarily representive of Chinese prostitution in general. The interviews were allowed only because the director wanted an explanation of their aggressive behavior, which occurred monthly, and was not typical of the institution's inmates. Yet their stories are excellent evidence that the revival of prostitution was not necessarily the result of the open-door policy and economic reform. For example, Ms. Zu left her family and became a street prostitute as early as 1971, well in advance of the first steps toward cultural openness and economic reform in 1979.

Ms. L. was 37 years old, married, and lived in a semirural district of Shanghai. Her husband frequently left home to work. She engaged in sex for pay with as many as three men a day, charging from 3 to 10 yuan (at that time, about U.S. $1.50 to $5.00). Her worst experience was with a customer who wanted vaginal-manual intercourse ("fisting"), and severely injured her vagina. She suffered from severe premenstrual ten-sion, which may have been partially responsible for her attacks on in-structors, which usually occurred just before she menstruated.

Ms. Zu was 26 years old, unmarried, and lived in Zhongming county, Shanghai province. She left home at 12 and lived on the streets of Shanghai city for the next fourteen years, until she was arrested. She had no home, no friends, no job. What she had was a medium-sized bag which held one change of clothing. She might sleep with one man for several days, or three men in one day. She got all her food, clothing, and shelter from these men. For the most part, she did not know their names and would not have recognized them if she met them again. By the time of the interview, she estimated that she had had sexual intercourse with more than 300 men. She said that once she had genuinely fallen in love with a young soldier and wanted to marry him. When she learned that her boyfriend's commanding officer would investigate her before grant-ing permission to marry, she was terrified and ran away. Now she was not only homeless again—she felt hopeless as well. She became very anxious and nervous, and began to suffer severe premenstrual tension. She said she needed a cold shower every day "to cool her heart."

Stories like those of Ms. L. and Ms. Zu represent the early, scattered beginnings of prostitution's revival in the 1970s. The very different story of the 1980s is one of rapid growth in the number of prostitutes, the profitability of the trade, and the level of its organization. Numerous statistics illustrate these changes.

The growth of prostitution in Kuangzhou (Canton) alone was amazing. In 1979 only 49 pimps, prostitutes, and customers were caught. In 1985, this number had increased to approximately 2,000. In one month of 1987—June—11,946 people were arrested for involvement in prostitution, and in both July and August the figures rose to more than 13,000 (Yi, 1988; Wen, 1988a).

Other statistics showed that in the 22 months from January 1985 to October 1987, more than 100,000 persons were found to be involved in prostitution. Prostitutes and their customers appeared everywhere—in hotels, inns, hair salons, single-family homes, apartments, dormitories, underground brothels, and taxis, in every city and every province. In the first seven months of 1987, there were 87% more arrests of prostitutes and their customers than in the same period of 1986 (Wen, 1988a). Between July and October of 1987, the rate of arrest of prostitutes and customers in all of China increased from 370% to 450%, depending on the location. Between January of 1986 and July of 1987, 18 prison camps for prostitutes were founded, and by December the number of camps—62—had more than tripled (author's translation from Du, Yi, & Xiong, 1988).

Statistics collected in 1986 in the city of Kuangzhou (Canton), in Kuangdong province supply some information about the men who patronize prostitutes. In 1986, of the 1,580 customers who were caught, 41% were from the city, 34.48% from the province, 15.3% from other provinces, 6.1% from Hong Kong and Macao, and 3.7% from other countries. Sixty-six customers were Communist Party members and county officials (Yi, 1988).

A typical example of the recent growth of prostitution in mainland China is the case of Changchun, the capital of Jilin province, a city which is not as large and open as Beijing, Shanghai, or Canton, but is much larger than many small cities and rural towns. A broad survey of prostitution in Changchun (which is called "C city" in the original formal publication) reported by Huai (1989) found that prostitution was far more active than it had been in 1949 before the founding of the People's Republic of China. In 1949, there were 23 registered brothels, 17 known illegal brothels, and a total of 316 known prostitutes. In 1988, after 40 years of the Communist government's strenuous efforts to eliminate prostitution, Changchun had a population of 1,800,000, and an estimated total of 1,000–1,500 prostitutes. Of the city's 1,000 private hotels, at least 250 hotels were involved in the daily transactions of about 250 prostitutes. Another 300 women were expensive "call girls," typically charging 300–500 yuan (about U.S. $80–135) a night. The highest prices were commanded by (presumed) virgins, who could charge 1,000 yuan (about U.S. $270). It was estimated that 70–80% of Changchun's prostitutes had sexually transmitted diseases (STD), primarily gonorrhea. The girl with the reputation of being the city's youngest prostitute was only thirteen years old (author's translation).

Gargan (1988) reports that when a woman is asked why she is a prostitute, she often replies simply, "I need money." There is no doubt that economic motives fuel the current rapid growth of prostitution in mainland China, and the country's leaders acknowledge this fact. The *World Journal* of July 2, 1990, reports a speech by Mr. Mei, the vice president of the People's Political Consultative Conference of Canton, stating that some prostitutes are members of the families of high officials, and some are even college students. Only the high pay could motivate women in these social positions to accept the risks attendant on prostitution.

THE CURRENT ATTEMPT TO SUPPRESS PROSTITUTION IN CHINA

In the late 1980s, even harsher measures were taken in the effort to curtail prostitution, including arrests of foreign citizens. For example, on September 8, 1987, the *Centre Daily News* reported an incident in which four Americans, one of whom was apprehended while in bed with a Chinese woman, were detained up to twelve hours by the Shanghai Police Department. Two of them were fined, one for 2,500 yuan and the other for 4,000 yuan (at that time, U.S. $1,078). Two days later, the same newspaper reported that a West German businessman had been fined 13,710 yuan (U.S. $3,695) after it was found that he had entertained a Chinese prostitute in his hotel room. It was also reported that prostitutes who sell their services to foreigners will be imprisoned for two years, with even longer terms for their pimps.

Similar measures were taken in other regions. In Canton, the police arrested more than 7,000 prostitutes in 1987. In June 1988, in the Shenzhen Economic Zone, which abuts Hong Kong, there was a mass arrest of 122 prostitutes and 100 customers, including Shenzhen policemen,

Communist Party officials, and Hong Kong truckers. In the small town of Deqing, about 100 miles west of Canton, a man accused of being a pimp was executed (Gargan, 1988).

There are three primary reasons for the redoubled attacks on prostitution:

1. There is a grave concern about the threat of sexually transmitted disease (STDs) to public health. In particular, the fear of AIDS is so extreme that it can fairly be described as "AIDS phobia." The Chinese government sees the elimination of prostitution as a vital part of any plan for controlling and preventing AIDS and other STDs.

China's Minister of Health, Dr. Min-zhang Chen, reported on August 5, 1989, at the National Symposium on AIDS Prevention Policy in Beijing, that China is one of the countries with the lowest reported incidence of AIDS in the world. He went on to say that the first case of AIDS discovered in China, in June, 1985, was that of an American tourist, and that as of August, 1989, only three cases of AIDS had been discovered. All three were infected abroad. Also, by July 27, 1989, only 26 cases of HIV infection had been diagnosed. The minister pointed out that in China, the only major mode of transmission of AIDS is through sexual contact. (In China, there is little IV drug use.) Yet, Dr. Chen warned, in recent years there had been a spread of venereal disease to every province and all the major cities (in mainland China the phrase "venereal disease" is still preferred to "sexually transmitted disease," and here the phrases VD and STD will be used interchangeably). Statistics had been gathered which showed that, in 16 major cities, the average incidence of VD was 21.02/100,000 in 1987, and in some the incidence was as high as 336/100,000, resembling that in some Western countries. Dr. Chen, emphasizing that prevention of sexual transmission was the key to controlling the spread of AIDS, enumerated several preventive strategies then in use: measures to prevent transmission of AIDS by visitors from abroad, a program to discover AIDS cases and HIV carriers as early as possible, and a general effort to control venereal diseases nationwide (*People's Daily*, August 6, 1989).

The following October, the first AIDS case in China was identified. The patient was a native Chinese citizen who sought medical care using an assumed name and was found to be suffering from secondary syphilis. The hospital later tested his blood serum and found it was HIV antibody positive. By the time the young man was identified, he had already left the country. (According to the head of the National AIDS Center, this patient said he had had homosexual relationships with foreigners.) Before this time, the Chinese government had found 24 foreigners and 1 person from Hong Kong carrying the AIDS virus. The first case of a native Chinese citizen with AIDS was seen as a dangerous signal for a country with such a large population. Beijing's public health authorities decided to expand AIDS testing to all VD patients and sexual offenders (*China Daily*, October 1989).

Whether or not prostitution is to blame, concern about STDs is well-founded. A public health problem that seemed to have been vanquished has assumed major proportions. In Helongjiang province alone, the incidence of VD increased at the rate of 8.9 times per year from 1982–1988. By the end of 1988, when this province had the fourth highest incidence in the country, 4,558 cases had been reported, and it was estimated that reported cases represented only 20% of the total incidence (*Centre Daily News*, July 15, 1989). Other local statistics on STDs are collected in Table 5–4. In China as a whole, the total number of VD cases reported from 1980 through the end of 1988 was 140,648, with more than 56,000 (over 39%) of these cases occurring in 1988 alone (World Journal, July 12, 1989).

2. The opposition to prostitution also has an ideological basis. In the lexicon of China's Communist leadership, "prostitution" is a very bad word. Deng Xiaoping, China's top leader, is particularly strong in his opposition to prostitution, which he believes tarnishes his country's reputation, and he advocates severe penalties.

It is also possible that China's leaders are embarrassed by the indictment of their economic policies represented by the continuing existence of prostitution. Considering that the Chinese Communist Party's earliest policy was to combat prostitution by offering women economic alternatives, it must be humiliating for them to hear that Chinese women

Table 5–4. Epidemiology of STDs in the People's Republic of China

Region surveyed	Gender/age/social distribution (% reported cases)	Disease distribution (% reported cases)	
16 major cities	Males 70% Females 30%	Gonorrhea	77.50%
		Syphilis	16.77%
		Others	5.73%
"A" Province		Syphilis	75%
		Others	5.73%
Jiangsu Province	More than 50% under 30 years old		
Shanghai	75% in the 20–34-year-old range	Gonorrhea	96%
	45% unmarried	Others	4%
	72% government employees		
	13% private businesspersons		
	15% otherwise employed		

Sources: *Centre Daily News*, January 24, 1989; March 10, 1989; April 28, 1989.

tell Western sociologists that they engage in prostitution because they need the money.

3. Vocal opposition to prostitution also results from political struggles within the CCP. Accusations of moral looseness are an effective means of silencing opposition, and each faction seeks not only to avoid criticism, but to be loudest in condemning "corruption."

Moreover, sexual repression is an important and effective element of the general strategy for controlling the life of the common people. While neither the conservative nor reform wings openly attacks other rights and freedoms, they are completely open in attacking the sexual freedom and the sexual rights of common people (including commercial sex). Thus in the wake of the Tiananmen Square massacre on June 4, 1989, China's new leaders accused Zhao, the former General Secretary of the CCP, of supporting commercial sex and "sex liberation," and included a drive against prostitution in the general increase of repression. Mass arrests of accused prostitutes and customers were made, and, whereas before the crackdown on the democracy movement only native Chinese patrons of prostitutes were sentenced to labor camp, it was announced in September 1989 by the new leader Li Ruihuan, one of the six top leaders and a standing member of the Politburo of the Chinese Communist Party Central Committee, that foreign nationals would be subject to the same sentence (*World Journal*, September 18, 1989). In Beijing, in the three weeks from November 25 to December 15, some 103 prostitutes were arrested (*World Journal*, December 26, 1989). According to the formal report by Yu Lei, the vice minister of the Department of Public Security of the People's Republic of China, during the antiprostitution, antipornography campaign initiated after the Tiananmen massacre, by January 15, 1990 there were arrests in more than 35,000 cases of prostitution involving more than 79,000 prostitutes and customers (*People's Daily*, February 10, 1990). Some of those arrested received sentences as severe as the death penalty.

For example, in Wenzhou city, Zhejiang province, a woman named Ni Pingfan and a man named Guan Wenchung were sentenced to death because, from September 1988 to September 1989, they had owned several underground brothels employing 14 prostitutes (*World Journal*, December 12, 1989). In Beijing a 55-year-old man named Ho Shuqi was given a death sentence because in 1988 he had allowed prostitutes to use the offices in Longtan Hospital more than 20 times. He was arrested for pandering on November 26, 1988 (*International Daily News*, January 22, 1990). This procurer was sentenced more than a year after his arrest; it was obvious that the sentence was intended as a show of strength in response to the embarrassment of the events at Tiananmen Square.

The latest politically motivated crackdown on prostitution, coupled with the parallel increase in censorship which will be described in the next chapter, suggests that public health concerns, however valid, are not the primary basis of antiprostitution policies. From that point of view, the government-controlled prostitution of the imperial and republican eras would be more sensible. It is obvious that people will not risk being sentenced to hard labor or death in order to seek medical care, and the increase in sexually transmitted infections is likely to continue. To the extent that government policies toward prostitution are a measure of the sexual freedom and well-being of the people, the situation in China is probably the worst it has ever been.

Chapter 6

Classical Chinese Erotica
Then and Now

CLASSIFICATIONS OF CHINESE FICTIONAL WORKS

China possesses one of the world's great literary traditions, with an uninterrupted history of more than 3,000 years. More than a thousand years ago, Chinese prose literature diverged into two streams. The first, more literary stream, known as classical prose, includes works emulating the standards and styles set by the authors of the Confucian Classics and the early philosophers. The language in such works is always far removed from contemporary dialects. By contrast, the second stream consists of vernacular prose, written in the same language their authors used on a daily basis. The same distinction exists in the realm of Chinese fiction.

Some scholars, including Chai and Chai (1965), Lu Hsun (1976), and Feng (1983), have categorized Chinese fiction according to the particular style of each work and the time at which it was written. According to this scheme, Chinese fiction falls into the following four categories:

1. Prose romances (Ch'uan-Ch'i, literally "transmission of the strange") mainly produced during the Tang dynasty (A.D. 618–907)
2. Story guides (Hua-Pen, literally "story-texts"), storytellers' scripts or prompt-books mainly recorded during the Sung, Yuan, and Ming dynasties (A.D. 960–1644)
3. Vernacular novels of the Ming and Ching Dynasties (A.D. 1368–1911)
4. Modern fictions written after the Literary Revolution of 1917

For our purposes, works in the first three of these categories constitute classical Chinese fiction.

Not all classical fictions are equally valuable as resources for the study of Chinese sexual behavior. The author has examined numerous works and scored them on a scale of 1–4 for their usefulness in sexological research. The Ruan Eroticism Scale is described below:

> 1. Fully erotic fiction: Works receiving this score consisted primarily or entirely of explicit sexual descriptions. An example is *The Prayer Mat of Flesh* (Jou Pu Tuan).
> 2. Partially erotic fiction: Works receiving this score include a considerable amount of explicit sexual description. An example is *The Golden Lotus* (Chin Ping Mei).
> 3. Incidentally erotic fiction: Works receiving this score contain only a small amount of explicit sexual description, which is incidental to the overall character of the novel. Examples are the famous *Dream of the Red Chamber* (Hung Lou Meng) and *The Water Margin of 120 Chapters* (Yi Bai Er Shi Hui Shiu Hu Chuan).
> 4. Nonerotic fiction: Works receiving this score contain no explicit sexual description. Examples are *Journey to the West*, also known as *Monkey* (Hsi Yu Chi), and *The Romance of the Three Kingdoms* (San Kuo Yen Yi).

Although some prose romances and story guides received Ruan Scale scores 2 or 3, vernacular novels of the Ming and Ching dynasties constitute the bulk of what may be described as "classical Chinese erotic fiction." Generally speaking, works in these categories would be those described as fully or partially erotic according to the Ruan Scale.

BIBLIOGRAPHIES OF CLASSICAL CHINESE EROTIC NOVELS

There are several bibliographies of classical Chinese vernacular novels (Sun Kaiti, 1958, 1982; Liu Cunren, 1982; Tan Chengpi, 1984). The most important is Sun Kaiti's *A Catalogue of Chinese Works of Popular Fiction* (Zhongguo tongsu xiaoshuo shumu), first published in 1932 and reprinted in 1958 and 1982. It is the only catalog of Chinese popular fiction which has a separate category for erotic fiction. This category is titled "weixie," which means "obscene" or "pornographic," and lists 42 books; it is the only published bibliography of classical Chinese erotic novels. The listing includes lost works and others that Sun has never seen personally. There are 33 currently extant novels included in Sun's bibliography, and these are listed in Table 6–1; we have added annotations indicating the editions in which these works are available.

Table 6–1. Sun's Listing of Classical Chinese Erotic Literature,
with Annotations

Period of origin	Title and author	Modern edition[a]
Ming dynasty (A.D. 1368–1644)	Xiu-ta ye-shi (*Unofficial Records of the Embroidered Couch*) by Lu Tien-Cheng (A.D. 1580–1620)	[A, C]
	Lang-shi (*Romantic Story*), Anonymous	[A, C]
	Bei-yuan-chuan (*One Hundred Love Stories*), Anonymous	[None]
	Shang-fung-chi (*Two Peaks Records*), Anonymous	[None]
	Chi-po-zi-chuan (*Life of the Foolish Woman*), Anonymous	[A, C]
Ching dynasty (1644–1911)	Jou Pu Tuan (*The Prayer Mat of Flesh*), Anonymous	[A, C] English translation available (Martin, 1967)
	Dang-yue-yuan (*The Predestined Relationship between the Lamp and the Moon*) by Xu Cheng	[None]
	Tao-hua-ying (*The Shadow of the Peach Blossom*) by Xu Cheng	[None]
	Nong-qing-kua-shi (*The Happy Story of Intense Passion*), Anonymous	[C]
	Wu-tung-ying (*The Shadow of a Chinese Parasol*), Anonymous	[None]
	Wu-shan-yan-shi (*The Merry Adventures of Wu-shan Mountain*), Anonymous	[A, C]
	Xing-hua-tian (*The Season of Apricot Blossom*), Anonymous	[None]
	Lian-qing-ren (*Longing for a Lover*), Anonymous	[None]
	Yu-fei mei-shi (*The Charming Story of the Imperial Concubine Named "Jade"*), Anonymous	[None]
	Dong you chi (*Journey to the East*), Anonymous	[B]
	Cui-shiao-mong (*Awakening in the Morning after Dreaming*), Anonymous	[None]
	Deng-cao He-shang (*The Biography of a Buddhist Monk Called Rush*), Anonymous	[A, C]
	Zhu-lin ye-shi (*Unofficial History of the Bamboo Garden*), Anonymous	[A, C]
Date unknown (Ming or Qing)	Tao-hua yan-shi (*The Merry Adventures of Peach Blossom*), Anonymous	[A, C]
	San miao chuan (*Three Wonderful Biographical Stories*), Anonymous	[A, C]

(*continued*)

Table 6–1. (continued)

Period of origin	Title and author	Modern edition[a]
	Kong-kong-huan (Empty, Empty, and Illusory), Anonymous	[None]
	Chun-deng mi-shi (The Fascinating Stories of the Spring Lanterns), Anonymous	[A, C]
	Hu-chun-ye-shi (Unofficial History of Appealing Spring), Anonymous	[None]
	Nao-hua-cong (Playing Around Among the Flowers), Anonymous	[C]
	Qi-yuan-ji (The Record of a Marvelous Predestined Relationship), Anonymous	[A]
	Shuang-yin-yuan (Pairs of Predestined Relationships), Anonymous	[None]
	Xiu-ge-pao-quan-chuan (The Fully Biographical Story of an Embroidered Military Uniform), Anonymous	[C]
	Feng-liu-he-shang (Loose Buddhist Monk), Anonymous	[None]
	Yan-hun-ye-shi (Unofficial History of Glorious Marriage), Anonymous	[None]
	Liao-qi-yuan (Settling the Marvelous Predestined Relationship), Anonymous	[None]
	Bi-yu-lou (Jasper Storied Building), Anonymous	[None]
	Cai-hua-xin (Picking the Heart of a Flower), Anonymous	[None]
	Zhao-yang qu-shi (The Interesting Story of the Imperial Consort Zhao Fei-yan), Anonymous	[A, C]

[a][A]: Text reprinted in its entirety in "Zhong-guo gu-yan xi-pingcong-kan" (Chinese Classical Erotic Rare Book Series, Tan-ch'ing Book Company, Taipei, Taiwan, 1986. This series included 44 titles in 22 volumes; some titles are nonfiction sexual books, including, for example, several famous Taoist handbooks of sexual technique.
[B]: Text partially reprinted in the above series.
[C]: Reprinted in "Ming-Qing Shan-ban shiao-shuo cong-kan: yan-qing shiao-shuo zuan-ji" (Ming-Qing Rare Fictions Series: Erotic Novels Series) by T'ien-yi Ch'u-pan-she, Taipei, Taiwan, 1985. This series included 25 titles in 37 volumes, all of them erotic fictions.

However, Sun's bibliography of erotic novels is incomplete in two respects. First, he listed some novels containing extensive erotic materials in categories other than "weixie"; second, some very rare erotic novels are not listed. Additional works which should be included in the category of classical Chinese erotic fictions are listed in Table 6–2.

It is important to note that many novels and short fictions which are not primarily erotic in character, some of them very famous, include passages containing very explicit and detailed descriptions of sexual be-

Table 6–2. Additional Examples of Classical Chinese Erotic Literature

Title and origin	Modern edition[a]
Nong-qing-kua-shi (*The Happy Story of Intense Passsion*) by Yun-ju shan-ren*	[A]
Yi-Chun Xiang-Zhi (*Pleasant Spring and Fragrant Character*) by Zuixifu Xinyuezhuren (pseudonym)	[C]
Bian er Chai (*Wearing a Cap but also Hairpins*) by Zuixifu Xinyezhuren (pseudonym)	[C]
Ru-yi-chun-chuan (*The Biography of Mr. "After-one's-own-heart"*), attributed to (Ming) Xu Changlin	[A, C]
Sui-Yang-ti yashi (*The Merry Adventures of Emperor Yang*), Anonymous	[None]
Seng-ni nie-hai (*Monks and Nuns in a Sea of Sins*), attributed to Tang yin	[A, C] English translation available. (Yang & Levy, 1971)
You Xian Ku (*The Fairies' Cavern*) by Chang Tsu (mainly active A.D. 679–715)	

*Same title as a book in Table 6–1, but different content.
[a][A]: Text reprinted in its entirety in "Zhong-guo gu-yan xi-pingcong-kan" (Chinese Classical Erotic Rare Book Series), Tan-ch'ing Book Company, Taipei, Taiwan, 1986. This series included 44 titles in 22 volumes; some titles are nonfiction sexual books, including, for example, several famous Taoist handbooks of sexual technique.
[B]: Text partially reprinted in the above series.
[C]: Reprinted in "Ming-Qing Shan-ban shiao-shuo cong-kan: yan-qing shiao-shuo zuan-ji" (Ming-Qing Rare Fiction Series: Erotic Novels Series) by T'ien-yi Ch'u-pan-she, Taipei, Taiwan, 1985. This series included 25 titles in 37 volumes, all of them erotic fiction.

havior. These materials are valuable sources of information about the sexual life of the classical era. These sources are listed in Table 6–3.

FICTIONAL DEPICTIONS OF SEXUAL BEHAVIOR

The old maxim asserting that there is nothing new under the sun may well be true of human sexual behavior. The author spent the years of 1984 and 1985 studying the collection of sexual art and literature in the Beilinshi Branch of the Beijing Library. (The Beilinshi Branch is a storage facility for one of the world's largest libraries; its collection includes many books which have been banned because of their explicit sexual descriptions and are unavailable elsewhere.) Studying this literature, I was repeatedly surprised to find descriptions of every imaginable sexual practice. Many behaviors which seemed entirely new (at the very least as subjects of open discussion), the apparent result of the sexual revolution that had taken place in the West in the 1960s and 1970s, ap-

Table 6–3. Selected Literary Sources of Erotic Descriptions

1.	Chin Ping Mei (*The Golden Lotus*)
2.	Yu-Shih Ming-Yen (*Stories for Enlightened Men*)
3.	Ching-Shih Dong-Yen (*Stories to Warn Men*)
4.	Hsin-Shih Heng-Yen (*Stories to Awaken Men*)
5.	P'o-an ching-ch'i (Pa-An Ching-Chi, *Striking the Table in Amazement at the Wonders*)
6.	Erh-k'o P'o-an ching-ch'i (Erh-Kuo Pa-an Ching-chi, *The Second Collection of Striking the Table in Amazement at the Wonders*)
7.	Hun-lou Meng (*Dream of the Red Chamber*)
8.	Ping-hua Bao-jan (*A Mirror of Theatrical Life*)
9.	Ye-shou Po-yan (*An Old Rustic's Idle Talk*)
10.	Hsing-Shih Yin-Yuan Chuan (*A Marriage to Awaken the World, or Lessons for Married Men*)
11.	Ch'an-Chen Hou-Shih (*The Later History of the Zen Master*)
12.	Nu-Xian Wai-Shi (*Romance of the Witch Tang Sai-erh*)

peared in the fragile, dusty scrolls dating from the late Ming and Ching dynasties (1500s to 1800s).

Besides portraying the most common marital sexual relationships and every possible position for sexual intercourse, the collection included descriptions and illustrations of a staggering variety of relationships and techniques which are only partially listed here (most of the explanations of sexual terminology are based on Kel & Ruan [1987]).

Of special sociological interest is the inclusion of tales featuring the sexual activities of Buddhist and Taoist monks and nuns. Since these individuals' religious status was supposed to require sexual abstinence, stories depicting them in sexual situations seem to have had an especially salacious quality, in the same way that European erotic literature from the Middle Ages through the Enlightenment sometimes featured sexually "corrupt" priests, monks, and nuns. The attempt to invoke the thrill of the forbidden may also have motivated depictions of incestuous, pedophilic, premarital, and adulterous (with or without spousal consent) relationships, and group sex ranging from threesomes to full-blown orgies.

A full range of erotic techniques is also represented in this literature. Thus male and female masturbation, the use of aphrodisiacs and mechanical sexual aids, oral and anal stimulation, including mutual oral-genital stimulation ("69"), and interfemoral intercourse are all to be found. Also found are such tender variations in love-play as erotic bathing and sensuous feeding. Frequently these behaviors are framed in a story line involving seduction or defloration.

Finally, statistically unusual and paraphiliac behaviors are broadly represented. Male and female homosexual relationships are portrayed in full and sympathetic detail, as is discussed in Chapter 7. Transvestism is discussed in Chapter 8. Exhibitionism and voyeurism, sadism and masochism, dominance and submission, fetishism (derivation of sexual gratification from nonsexual body parts or objects), necrophilia (sexual interaction with corpses), urophilia (sexual arousal from urinating on another person or being urinated on), planned and impulsive rape are all to be found.

One of the difficulties of identifying sexual themes and behaviors in erotic fiction is that some categories overlap; for example, incest and group sex necessarily involve nonmarital sex, and defloration can occur within marriage. A detailed study of the sexological substance of classical Chinese fictions is an immense task beyond the scope of this chapter. Instead, some excerpts of erotic fiction are given as examples. These examples also demonstrate how a content analysis of such sources can yield the type of information discussed above. Analyses are in parentheses.

Unofficial History of the Bamboo Garden (Zhu-lin ye-shi)

This novel is a historical fiction set in the "Spring and Autumn Period" (770–476 B.C.) of the Zhou dynasty. The major character, Princess Su'e, the daughter of King Mu (reigned 627–606 B.C.) of the state of Zheng, is presented as a very lustful, sexually adept woman. Upon reaching puberty, she has a dream in which she meets with a Taoist adept, who initiates her into the secrets of sexual intercourse. This dream is the beginning of Su'e's amorous career. She begins by seducing a young cousin, then having her maid, Hehua, join them in a menage à trois (premarital sex, group sex, incest).

Soon after, Su'e is married to the son of a neighboring king, King Ling of Chen. The novel describes her amorous play with her husband in a bamboo grove in the palace gardens. Before long Su'e gives birth to a son, and soon afterward her husband dies of exhaustion; on his deathbed he entrusts his widow and infant son to a close friend, the Minister Kong Ning.

Su'e has sexual relations with both Kong and another minister, Yi Xingfu (adultery). In order to safeguard his own position, Kong arranges a meeting between Su'e and her father-in-law, King Ling. To give the king the greatest possible pleasure, Su'e has him lie on his back, then mounts him, moving her vagina up and down on his penis "like a small mouth eating a cherry," giving him an intense orgasm (incest, adultery, woman-superior position).

Now the king also joins in the sexual orgies in the Bamboo Grove, in which Su'e's maid, Hehua, continues to take an active part. There are numerous descriptions of group sex among various combinations of characters. In one passage, Minister Yi drinks wine from a cup placed between Su'e's thighs (sensuous feeding, eating, or drinking).

Twenty years pass; Su'e and Hehua still look like young girls, but their lovers have grown old and weak (this example of mystical sexuality is the result of Taoist sexual practices which some have described as "sexual vampirism"). One day, Su'e's son, who has grown to be a strong warrior, overhears the king and his two ministers jokingly speculating as to which of them is his father. Infuriated, he attacks and kills the king. The two ministers escape and take refuge in the enemy state of Chu. King Zhuang of Chu, having long planned to attack Chen, now uses the murder of King Ling as a pretext. Su'e's son is killed in battle and she herself is taken captive and separated from her maid Hehua.

At the court of Chu there is a minister, Qu Wu, who is an expert in methods of strengthening the vital essence by sexual intercourse. He wants to marry Su'e, but King Zhuang has her married to an elderly general. About a year later, after her husband's death in battle, Su'e and her stepson Hedui seduce each other and enjoy each other tremendously. One night, Su'e pretends to rape Hedui, using the woman-superior position while he pretends to be in a deep sleep (fantasy play, incest).

Eventually Qu Wu succeeds in getting a promotion and marrying Su'e. Their sexual life is wonderful. On one occasion, they enjoy themselves so much that a maid who overhears them becomes aroused (ecouteurism) and convinces another servant to take her virginity in a scene which even describes her bleeding in detail (seduction, defloration).

Meanwhile, the maid Hehua, who had avoided capture, begins a sexual relationship with a young man even before his parents grant them permission to marry (premarital intercourse). Then, after her husband is murdered by robbers, Hehua is reunited with Su'e. Su'e's husband Qu takes Hehua as a concubine, and the three enjoy many sexual encounters (menage à trois). Qu, Su'e, and Hehua, as expert practitioners of Taoist sexual disciplines, need young partners to supply them with vital essence. Qu Wu succeeds in convincing the young nobleman Liangshu and his wife to join them in their orgies (adultery, group sex). Thus the Bamboo Grove is reestablished in Chin. Eventually a servant betrays the orgiasts to the king, who has his soldiers surround Qu Wu's mansion. Liangshu and his wife are arrested, but Su'e, Hehua, and Qu Wu have already absorbed so much vital essence that they have completed their "Inner Elixir." Now immortals, they disappear into the sky shrouded by a cloud of mist.

The Prayer Mat of Flesh (Jou Pu Tuan)

In the Chinese edition, this novel begins with a discussion of the author's sexual philosophy which, unfortunately, was omitted in the Western translation. The author asserted that heterosexual intercourse is essential to a long and healthy life and a source of pleasure which relieves everyday sorrows. He argued that court eunuchs and most Buddhist monks were short-lived because they did not engage in sexual intercourse. A large part of the novel is a dramatic presentation of the contrasts between sex-positive and sex-negative viewpoints, in which the hero extols sexual pleasure and his wife in the beginning advocates conservatism and prudery.

The hero is a young, talented scholar named Wei-yang-sheng (the Before-Midnight Scholar). Both his relationship with his principal wife Yu Xiang (Jade Perfume, or Noble Scent) and his sexual adventures with six other women are described in the course of the novel.

Wei-yang-sheng's bride is the daughter of a well-known literary scholar. Her father has given her a good literary education, but supervised her so strictly that she is very naive. Although beautiful, she is extremely reserved and completely ignorant of sexual matters, making the ardent young man feel that he was deceived into marrying her. The young husband's frustration is graphically portrayed: If he makes a sexual remark, his wife blushes and runs away. He prefers to make love during the day, so he can be aroused by the sight of his wife's genitals; but whenever he approaches her before dark, she protests as loudly as if he were a rapist. At night, she makes it clear that she is accepting his advances only because she has no choice.

The descriptions of Wei-yang-sheng's attempts to make intercourse pleasurable provide a clear picture of what was considered acceptable in marital intercourse and the language in which it was described. He tries to introduce various positions: First he attempts "to catch the fire across the mountain" (rear entry), but Jade Perfume protests that it is wrong for a wife to turn her back on her husband. When he suggests that they "moisten the inverted candle" (assume the woman-superior position), she argues that doing so would invert the correct position of the male and female principles. It takes a considerable effort even to persuade her to place her feet on his shoulders. She never utters the usual exclamations meant to compliment a man's sexual prowess, such as "You kill me!" or "My life!" and is totally unresponsive to her husband's endearments.

Wei-yang-sheng finally decides that his only hope is to give his wife the sexual education she never received. He goes to an antique shop and purchases an album of very fine erotic paintings by a famous artist. The album consists of thirty-six paintings, each corresponding to a line in the Tang poem "Spring Reigns in All the Thirty-six Palaces." He hopes that when Jade Perfume sees the paintings, she will realize that the sexual variations he has suggested are not his own inventions, but have in fact been practiced since ancient times.

When Jade Perfume opens the album to the first page, she sees written in large characters, "Lingering Glory of the Han Palace," and assumes that she will see portraits of the wise empresses and chaste ladies of that ancient time. When she turns the page to a painting of a nude couple in a sexual embrace, she is shocked and embarrassed and wants to burn the book. Wei-yang-sheng stops her, telling her the book is a valuable antique that he has borrowed from a friend, and she should not burn it unless she is prepared to pay a hundred silver pieces in compensation.

There follows a long argument which is clearly the vehicle for explaining the author's sexual philosophy. Jade Perfume asks, "What is the use of looking at such an unorthodox thing?" Her husband replies, "If this were really such an unorthodox thing, then why should the artist have painted it?" adding, "... this album represents the most orthodox thing which has existed since the creation of the universe." He points out that such albums are sold in many antique shops, that they grace the libraries of connoisseurs and eminent scholars, and that they are a means of transmitting ancient knowledge about the best way to conduct a marriage. Without them, he says, "Husbands would abandon their spouses and wives turn their backs on their men. The line of creation would be broken off and mankind would disappear." Reminding her that her father's only fear is that their union will not produce grandchildren, he argues that any knowledge leading to the conception of children "certainly belongs to the study of the Right Way!"

At first Jade Perfume is unconvinced, arguing that if sexual "antics" were proper, people would engage in them in daylight and in public. However, her husband insists that her attitude simply demonstrates that she is ignorant because her father was too overprotective to even allow her to discuss romance with her girlfriends. Finally, she agrees to sit in his lap and inspect the album with him. The album is unusual in that each painting is accompanied by a commentary discussing its artistic merits and erotic implications. Wei-yang-sheng reads each commentary aloud, hoping to arouse his wife and to inspire her to try what she sees in the pictures.

The narrative includes the text of five of these commentaries. One picture, "Posture of the Two Dragons Tired of the Fight," depicts a couple resting after orgasm: "The woman's head rests on the pillow, her arms lie by her side limp like a strand of silk...their souls seem to have left their bodies and now they are on the way to beautiful dreams." The commentary praises the subtlety of the artist, pointing out that the couple are so relaxed that they might seem dead, if it were not for the painter's skill in conveying the idea that in the ecstasy of orgasm, the man and woman seem to die together. (This appears to be a transcultural image—consider the French description of orgasm as "the little death.") At long last, Jade Perfume's passion is aroused. Just as Wei-yang-sheng is about to show her another painting, she pushes the album away, exclaiming, "What is the good of this book? It only hinders people when getting up. Look at it yourself, I am going to bed!"

From that time on Jade Perfume becomes increasingly passionate. The novel describes a number of erotic scenes between Jade Perfume and Wei-yang-sheng, as well as his sexual adventures with other women.

The novel's ending seems strangely at odds with the author's vigorous defense of human sexuality in the opening chapter. Perhaps, like the authors of some Western erotic literature, he punishes his hero to pacify more straitlaced critics, offering a "moral" that is actually an excuse for the telling of his tale. Eventually, Wei-yang-sheng's infidelities get him into serious trouble, and at the end of the novel he enters a monastery as a broken man and becomes a devout Buddhist. The abbot explains to him that for him, debauchery had been the necessary path to realizing the need for enlightenment. He has reached salvation by "the prayer mats of the flesh."

The Golden Lotus (Chin Ping Mei)

This novel uses a vigorous, colloquial language to recount the life of Hsi-men Ch'ing, the wealthy owner of a large pharmacy. In the course of the novel, he has 19 sexual partners, including his six wives. The novel contains 105 references to sexual intercourse, including 72 more or less detailed, explicitly sexual passages, many of them describing very novel practices (Zhu Xing, 1980). Some of the more unusual scenes are described here; in these descriptions, the name of one of Hsi-men's favorite wives is abbreviated as Chin.

In one passage, Hsi-men suspends the naked Chin upside down by tying her feet to a grape trellis, a position that opens her vagina very wide. First he has intercourse with her, using his hands to support her body. Then he throws plums into her vagina, later removing them and having her eat them (unusual position, sensuous feeding).

In another passage, when copious sexual secretions flow from a lover's vagina, she stops Hsi-men from wiping it up and eats it all (extramarital sex, sensuous eating). Then she asks him to insert his penis into her anus (anal intercourse), explaining that this is the only way she can achieve orgasm.

On one occasion, when Chin remains unsatisfied after intercourse, she sucks Hsi-men's penis all through the night (oral-genital contact), and finally asks him to urinate in her mouth, swallowing all the urine (urophilia). In a later chapter, Hsi-men tells another lover, "Chin loved me so much she drank my urine," and she replies, "I would like to do the same thing for you."

Additional passages describe the use of numerous sex toys and aphrodisiacs, different positions for intercourse, and oral and anal intercourse.

SUPPRESSION OF EROTIC FICTION IN THE YUAN, MING, AND CHING DYNASTIES (A.D. 1271–1911)

As noted in previous chapters, China's culture during the first 4,000 years of her recorded history was generally characterized by open and positive sexual attitudes. Then about a thousand years ago, during the Sung dynasty, sexual attitudes began to change, gradually becoming more and more negative and repressive. The crucial change was initiated by several famous Neo-Confucianists, including Chou Tun-i (1017–1073), Cheng Hao (1032–1085) and Cheng I (1033–1107), the founders of Neo-Confucianism, and Chu Hsi (1130–1200) who, as the major interpreter and systematizer, was the true father of Neo-Confucianism (T. Y. Chen, 1928; Harrison, 1972; van Gulik, 1961).

Cheng I summarized the Neo-Confucian viewpoint in a remark contained in his *Posthumous Papers*—"Discard human desires to retain the heavenly principles." When asked whether it was justifiable for a widow to remarry when pressed by poverty and hunger, he replied, "It is a very small thing to die as a result of starvation, but a very serious evil to lose chastity toward one's dead husband by remarrying" (T. Y. Chen, 1928; Xia, 1980).

Chu Hsi repeatedly emphasized his agreement with Cheng I. For example, Chu Hsi wrote a letter to his friend Cheng Shizhong urging him not to permit his widowed sister to remarry, justifying his viewpoint by quoting Cheng I's opinion, which he described as an unchangeable principle (Chen, T. Y., 1928). Chu Hsi's strictly Confucianist interpretation of the Classics was more rigorous than any that had gone before. He stressed the inferiority of women and the strict separation of the sexes, and forbade any manifestation of heterosexual love outside of wedlock. This narrow attitude is especially manifest in his commentaries on the love songs of the *The Book of Poetry* (described in Chapter 2), which he reinterprets as political allegories.

Chu Hsi laid the foundations of Neo-Confucianism as the sole state religion. It encouraged a strictly authoritarian form of government, including the establishment of censorship and thought control.

This trend was strengthened during the succeeding dynasty, the Yuan (1271–1368), which was founded and sustained by Mongol invaders. One of the major problems faced by the Chinese as an occupied nation was to protect their women from seduction or coercion by the conquerors. In this context, the Neo-Confucianist rules requiring the seclusion of women seemed quite desirable. Some scholars believe that it was these circumstances that gave rise to the prudery and secretiveness toward outsiders that have come to be characteristics of Chinese culture (van Gulik, 1961). In this period, erotic fiction was not sufficiently developed to attract official attention. However, the government banned any performance of plays or songs with erotic content at local fairs. The punishment was flogging: Performers were sentenced to 47 blows with a bamboo rod, organizers and fair managers were sentenced to 27 blows (Wang Liqi, 1981).

In 1422, during the early Ming dynasty, the central government banned all works that could be held to resemble *New Tales Written While Trimming the Wick* (Chien-teng hsin-hua), a prose romance published in 1378 which included some erotic stories. The government order stated that all copies of such books were to be burned, and anyone who printed, sold, collected, or read banned books was subject to punishment (Wang Liqi, 1981).

In 1664, twenty years after the founding of the Ching Dynasty, Emperor Kang-hsi (reigned A.D. 1661–1722) announced yet another ban on erotic literature. The government's list of banned books contained more than 150 titles, most of them erotic fictions (some other books were banned for their political content). In later versions of the laws of the Great Ching, there was a requirement that not only all copies of banned books but also the original woodblocks be burned. Harsh punishments were prescribed for anyone who published, distributed, or possessed banned literature. For example, a commoner or soldier involved in printing a banned book was beaten and exiled. Numerous lists of banned books were published during the Ching dynasty. Several complete lists are still extant. The contents changed little from one list to the next, though some were more extensive than others. Most of the banned books were erotic fictions, and nearly all the books listed in Table 6–1 were banned at one time or another (Wang Liqi, 1981).

The repeated bannings and burnings of woodblocks and manuscripts were all too successful; many of the classical works of erotic fiction are completely lost. In other cases, there exist only a very few copies which were secretly preserved in private collections. Some of the works still available to us (again, there are often only one or two copies) are in collections in Japan, the United States, England, France, and other locations outside China. This situation presents serious impediments to scholarship. For example, there is only one copy of the original editions of the very famous Ming short-story collections *The Two Strikes* (Erh-p'o), *Striking the Table in Amazement at the Wonders and The Second Collection of Striking the Table in Amazement at the Wonders,* edited by Ling Mengchu and published in 1628 and 1632. Both reprinted editions in mainland China, one published in 1957 and the other in 1982, were based on those collections, and to prepare them, the editors had to use a photocopy of a manuscript kept in a Japanese collection (Ling, 1982a, b). Even so, the modern reprints are incomplete: because of the current antipornography policy in mainland China, all erotic passages were omitted from both editions. Thus a thorough study of this special body of literature will require both a considerable investment of resources and relaxation of governmental censorship.

The censorship policy of the government of the Republic of China was inconsistent. Sometimes restrictions were relaxed, sometimes they were tightened, but there were always some restrictions on erotic literature. Nonetheless, reprinted copies of Ming and Ching erotica never really stopped circulating underground, and new works were written and published. However, modern works are not considered here, as their social impact has been less than that of the classical literature, they have less literary value and sexological interest, and are generally considered less important than the classical works.

THE COMPLETE PROHIBITION OF EROTICA IN MAINLAND CHINA TODAY

After the founding of the People's Republic of China on October 1, 1949, a strict ban on erotic fiction and sexually explicit materials of any kind was imposed nationwide. The "Rules for the Control of and Punishments Concerning Public Security of the People's Republic of China" (October 22, 1957) contain an article regarding punishment for persons accused of involvement with pornography:

> Article 5: A person who commits any of the following acts disrupting public order shall be punished by detention of not more than ten days, a fine of not more than twenty yuan, or a warning:

7. Putting up for sale or rent reactionary, obscene, or absurd books, periodicals, picture books, or pictures that have previously been repressed.

In the 1950s and 1960s, the policy of banning erotica was very effective. In the whole country, almost no erotic material was to be found. There were few difficulties implementing this policy until the mid-1970s. Then, the legalization and wide availability of erotica in several Western countries during the late 1960s and early 1970s, coupled with China's increasing openness to the outside world, increased the supply of such material available for underground circulation. In recent years, the suppression of pornography has become a very serious political and legislative concern. The number of arrests and the severity of sentences on people involved in pornography have both increased in the attempt to suppress it entirely.

To understand the current situation, it is necessary to review events during and after the "Cultural Revolution." During the late 1950s and early 1960s, the means of communication were completely nationalized; the print media, the broadcast media, and even bookstores and photographic studios were strictly controlled, and before the Cultural Revolution pornography was simply unavailable. By the middle of the Cultural Revolution, in about 1974, several hand-copied erotic short novels were secretly but broadly circulated, primarily among the youth—in high schools, colleges, and universities, and in factories. A typical example was the well-known *The Heart of a Young Girl* (also known as *The Memoir of Manna*), which is described in this chapter. The Chinese Communist Party (CCP) and the government captured many of these hand-copied booklets in different places across the nation by threatening to punish those who did not turn them over to authorities.

By the late 1970s, "XXX-rated" films and videotapes were being smuggled into China from Hong Kong and other countries. (In China, these are known as "yellow videos"; just as "blue movie" refers to erotic films in the United States, "yellow" refers to erotica in China.) Yellow videos quickly became a fad. At first the only people who could view these tapes were rather highly placed party members and their families, since only they had access to videotape players, which were very rare and expensive in China at that time. Before long, however, yellow videos, including the well-known American pornographic movie *Deep Throat*, were available to more people, although still very secretly and only through small underground circles. Some people used the tapes to make money; tickets for video shows were very expensive, usually 5–10 yuan per person (at that time most people's monthly salary was only about 40–50 yuan). Sometimes people who were watching these tapes engaged in sexual activity, even group sex. Because yellow videos were usually shown in small private rooms to very small audiences whose members knew each other well, a festive atmosphere often prevailed. It was very easy for young people to initiate sexual activity when they were aroused by what they saw.

At about the same time, erotic photographs, reproductions of paintings, and books were also smuggled into mainland China. They, too, were sold at a great profit. One small card with a nude photo would cost as much as 5 or 10 yuan.

There was a strong reaction at the highest levels of the CCP and the government. The police were ordered to confiscate every type of pornographic material, from hand-copied books to "yellow" audiotapes and films. Severe penalties were ordered for all people involved in the showing or viewing of "yellow" videos, and in April 1985 a new antipornography law was promulgated.

The new law was an administrative law, "The State Council's Regulations on Severely Banning Pornography." In addition to prohibiting every imaginable type of erotic material, it imposed much more severe penalties than those called for by the "Rules on...Public Security" of 1957. According to the new regulations:

> Pornography is very harmful, poisoning people's minds, inducing crimes...and must be severely banned. The items which must be severely banned include: any kind of video-tape, audio-tape, film, TV program, slide, photograph, painting, book, newspaper, magazine, and hand-copied material which contains explicit descriptions of sexual behavior and/or erotic pictures; any kind of toy or article with instructions for use which were printed above erotic pictures; and any kind of aphrodisiacs and sex-toys. The person who smuggled, produced, sold, or organized the showing of pornography, whether for sale or not, shall be punished according to the conditions, by imprisonment or administrative punishment.

In July of 1987, The State Council enacted even stricter antipornography policies. As we will discuss, these laws are enforced in an extremely repressive manner. Their use as an instrument of political repression is facilitated by the vagueness of the concept of "pornography." The definition is very loose and quite confusing, as the following cases illustrate.

In 1985, the author of this book, in his special capacity as a sex researcher, received special permission from a large urban police department to read confiscated erotic literature. A typical example was *The Heart of a Young Girl*, a short novel consisting of about 6,000 Chinese characters, which, as was earlier noted, circulated in handwritten copies and enjoyed considerable popularity. The novel, a simple love story describing the romance between the 18-year-old Manna and her cousin Xu, contains explicit, but not detailed, descriptions of premarital sex. The sexual behaviors mentioned include nude petting outdoors, penile-vaginal intercourse indoors, erotic bathing, and fellatio and cunnilingus—all rather tame by Western standards.

Two state-run publishing houses, the Beijing-based Workers' Publishing House and Yanbian People's Printing House in Jilin Province, were fined 600,000 and 400,000 yuan respectively (about U.S. $150,000 and $100,000) for distributing Chinese editions of *Gambler* and *Fun Club*, both translated from English editions. They were printed in editions of 370,000 copies and 400,000 copies, respectively. All copies were ordered destroyed, as well as the printing plates, and all profits were confiscated. The leading officials at the two publishing houses were disciplined. These two books, one by a British writer and another by an American writer, were labeled pornography by the authorities during the current nationwide drive against pornographic publications. The books were described as "full of pornographic content," "likely to encourage people to commit crimes," and "seriously harmful to young people, mentally and physically" (*China Daily*, July 13, 1988). By Western standards, these are mainstream novels which nobody would classify as "adult" or "erotic."

In June of 1988, the head of the Central Government Department of Publications, which controls all publications in China, ordered the banning of the *Story of Chin Ping Mei* (an abridgment of the famous novel Chin Ping Mei, known in English as *The Golden Lotus*), which had been produced by the Writers' Publishing House, a prestigious state-run literary publisher. The original edition of Chin Ping Mei, published in A.D. 1617, consists of over 1,000,000 characters, with about 30,000 characters (less than 3%) describing sexual behavior; the abridged edition, consisting of only 170,000 characters, contains no sexual descriptions at all. The decision to condemn the reproduced classic as "pornography," merely because it bears the title of a novel which originally contained explicit sex scenes, is simply ridiculous. The editor in chief of Writers' Publishing House, the famous author Cung Wi-xi, was so upset that he wrote a long article criticizing and protesting this absurd decision (*Centre Daily News*, June 28, 1988). One cannot help suspecting that the ban was motivated by some personal or professional animosity.

The suppression of materials labeled as pornographic was active and effective. In 1987, the deputy director of the National Publication Bureau announced that during the preceding three years 217 illegal publishers had been arrested. In the year ending in August 1986, 42 publishing houses had been forced to close. Most publishers received warnings and/or fines; one who had made a profit of 600,000 yuan (about U.S.

$200,000) in three years was sentenced to three years in prison (*Centre Daily News*, August 21, 1987). The nationwide crackdown on pornography led to numerous arrests and confiscations in city after city. For example, the Overseas Edition of the *People's Daily* reported on July 17, 1987, that in Beijing during the six previous weeks, three publishers of pornography had been detained and 60,000 books confiscated. Two weeks later the same publication announced that the Shanghai police had demanded the surrender of all pornographic materials, and readied a police force of thousands to arrest publishers of pornography. By October 15, 1987, the Shanghai police had confiscated 110,000 books and more than 5,000 video- and audiotapes (*Centre Daily News*, October 15, 1987). Also in July of 1987, the Fuzhou police and cultural departments began confiscating materials ranging from playing cards and calendars with nude illustrations to "yellow" videotapes; by the end of the first week of this campaign, more than 20,400 erotic pictures had been burned (*People's Daily*, Overseas Edition, August 2, 1987). Perhaps the most massive arrests of 1987 occurred in Nanchang, the capital of Jiangxi Province, where by October, 44 dealers in pornography had been arrested and 80,000 erotic books and magazines confiscated. It was reported that an underground publishing house with 600 salesmen had been circulating erotic materials in 23 of China's 28 provinces, making a profit of 1,000,000 yuan (in that period about U.S. $300,000) in two years (*Centre Daily News*, October 5, 1987).

Two incidents are especially noteworthy. The first involved a high-ranking official, Zhou Erfu, the author of the well-known novel *The Morning of Shanghai* and the biographical novel *Doctor Norman Bethune,* and former deputy minister of the Cultural Ministry of the State Council. In February 1986, he was dismissed from the position of vice president of the Association for Foreign Friendship and expelled from the CCP for having visited a sex shop and patronized a prostitute while on an official visit to Japan in late 1985 (*People's Daily*, Overseas Edition, March 4, 1986; *World Journal*, February 19, 1986).

In the second incident, a Shanghai railway station employee, Qinxiang Liang, was sentenced to death. Liang and four other persons organized sex parties on nine different occasions; during these parties they showed pornographic videotapes and engaged in sexual activity with female viewers. The other organizers were sentenced to prison, some for life (*Centre Daily News*, August 25, 1987).

The climax of this wave of repression seemed to occur on January 21, 1988, when the 24th Session of the Standing Committee of the 6th National People's Congress adopted supplemental regulations imposing stiffer penalties on dealers in pornography. Under these regulations, if the total value of the pornographic materials is between 150,000 yuan and 500,000 yuan, the dealer shall be sentenced to life imprisonment (*Centre Daily News*, January 23, 1988). But then Deng Xiaoping, China's top leader, went further by declaring that some publishers of erotica deserved the death penalty! (*Centre Daily News*, August 24, 1988.) It may be at least one of the most severe political punishments against "pornography" suggested by a national leader anywhere in the world.

Chinese Communist leaders seek to justify their position by claiming that pornography causes crime. For example, they cite a survey finding that of 689 juvenile delinquents, 65.9% had read handwritten "yellow" literature (of these 454 cases, 232 were male and 222 female). Of the female delinquents, 95% had read such literature. The author of the survey, using the statistics given in Table 6–4, sought to show a connection between the reading of pornography and sexual activity.

However, the political motives for this position are obvious. Like the campaign against prostitution, the campaign against pornography was redoubled in intensity after the massacre at Tiananmen Square on June 4, 1989. At that time, leaders of the conservative faction blamed the ousted Chinese Communist Party's leader Zhao Ziyang for the wide circulation of pornographic works in mainland China, and the new leaders vociferously attacked pornography. The *China Daily* of September 15, 1989 reported a typical statement by Li Ruihuan, one of the six top leaders, a Standing Member of the Politburo of the CCP Central Committee, saying he "pointed out that the antipornography drive is significant in relation to the focus on opposing bourgeois liberalization." This is the viewpoint of a man widely considered to represent the reform faction.

In the latest nationwide move against pornography, beginning on the thirty-seventh day after the Tiananmen Square massacre, on July 11,

Table 6–4. Sexual Relationships of Minors Convicted of Reading Pornography

Relationship	Male (232 cases)	Female (222 cases)
Has at least one intimate heterosexual friend	60.35% (140 cases)	90.99% (202 cases)
Has two or more intimate heterosexual friends[a]	41.38% (96 cases)	74.77% (166 cases)
Has five or more intimate heterosexual friends	No data given	36.48% (81 cases)
Has or had sexual intercourse with at least one partner	No data given	82.88% (184 cases)
Has or had sexual intercourse with three or four partners	No data given	29.73% (66 cases)

[a]May or may not have had sexual intercourse.
Source: Based on Yang, 1988.

1989, 65,000 policemen and other bureaucrats were mobilized to investigate publishing houses, distributors, and booksellers. By August 21, more than 11 million books and magazines had been confiscated and about 2,000 publishing and distributing centers and 100 private booksellers were forced out of business (*International Daily News*, August 24, 1989). To say the least, China's leadership must be aware that activity on this scale significantly impairs the flow of communication—and potential criticism—at a time of great social instability.

In the ensuing months, as the "antipornography" campaign was waged ever more relentlessly, political and ideological motivations continued to be apparent in Li Ruihuan's speeches. On October 17, 1989, in a report of a speech he had delivered the previous month urging the leaders of China's southern coastal provinces to make greater efforts, the *China Daily* quoted him as again describing the antipornography effort as part of the struggle against bourgeois liberalization. In both this speech and another reported in the English supplement to the *Sing Tao International* of February 13, 1990, Li asserted that "Hostile overseas forces have taken pornography, gambling, and drugs as a means of corroding the fighting will of the people," intentionally "tak[ing] advantage of the development of the reform and opening to the outside world to infiltrate with pornography."

Not only did China's leadership use their antipornography crusade as a means of asserting control of the communications media and engendering hostility against forces for liberalization, but they clearly hoped to quell prodemocracy sentiment. Thus Li Ruihuan, in his September 1989 speech, said the campaign was an effort to "help people to develop into a new type with high ideals...and a strong sense of morality and discipline."

Finally, the antipornography crusade has served as a means of coordinating and consolidating the present leaders' control over the apparatus of government. In his 1990 address, Li claimed that a successful effort must involve the departments of propaganda, culture, publishing, industry, commerce, taxation, public security, customs, border security, and education, as well as various mass organizations. Similarly, Zhao Dongming, head of the Beijing municipal group in charge of screening the publications market, said that their confiscation efforts in the autumn of 1989 involved coordinating the work of "inspectors from departments of industry and commerce, public security, publication and culture" (*China Daily*, November 27, 1989).

It is impossible to predict how far the CCP and the Chinese government will go in their battle against pornography. What is clear is that all Chinese political leaders, whether they belong to the reformist faction, the neutral faction, or the conservative faction, consistently oppose both pornography and prostitution, at least in public. Each group strives to outdo the others in its condemnations of "this kind of capitalist atrocity." The reformist faction is especially loud in its denunciations as it seeks to defend itself from conservative claims that the "open-door policy" is to blame for the introduction of such "rotten, decayed, corrupt, degenerating" phenomena.

The real victims of these policies are not the supposed villains whom the government accuses of preying on the Chinese people, but the people themselves. Either the government's claims of confiscating huge amounts of erotic materials are inflated or they refute the government's other claim that the antipornography crusade is born of the moral indignation of the populace. It seems more likely that the high price of erotic materials reflects the popular hunger for sex information that is described in the last chapter of this book. In any case, it is a very real possibility that the fierce attacks on the communications media will actually hinder China's modernization.

The "antipornography" campaign is more dangerous than the prudery and restrictiveness of neo-Confucian laws and customs. Anyone is vulnerable to arrest if it is merely reported that s/he possesses erotic materials, and the government policy of leniency to those who confess, and harshness to those who do not, is well known. In this atmosphere of suspicion, in which the elimination of "dangerous" literature about human sexuality is a cover for suppression of personal and political freedom, nobody can feel safe. Perhaps most tragically, human sexuality, and the pleasure and intimacy it creates, can hardly be expected to flourish.

Chapter 7

Homosexuality
From Golden Age to Dark Age

MALE HOMOSEXUALITY

Male homosexuality may have been a familiar feature of Chinese life in prehistoric times. The eminent Ching dynasty scholar Chi Yun cited an opinion in his famous *Notes of the Yue-Wei Heritage* that the position of "catamite" (a young male who serves as the lovemaking partner of an adult homosexual or bisexual) originated during the reign of the mythical Yellow Emperor, about 46 centuries ago (Ruan & Tsai, 1987). In any case, China's earliest historical records contain accounts of male homosexuality.

Probably the earliest record of homosexuality dates from the Shang (or Yin) dynasty (approximately the sixteenth to eleventh centuries B.C.). An ancient text, *The Historical Book of the Shang Dynasty,* contains the phrase "pi wangtong," which is translated as "having an intimate relationship with a catamite" (Pan, 1947).

Special Terms for Homosexuality in China

Before surveying the historical materials concerning homosexuality in ancient China, we will single out the three most famous historical incidents concerning Chinese homosexuals. Each of these stories is the source of one of the widely used colloquial terms for homosexuality.

The first story was recorded in "The Difficulties of Persuasion" in *Han Fei Tzu*, the works of the famous philosopher Han Fei who died in 233 B.C. The story concerns a king in the state of Wei named Ling (534– 493 B.C.), who was in love with a very handsome man called Mi Tzuhsia. According to the law of Wei, anyone who drove the king's carriage without permission would be punished by amputation of his legs. One day Mi Tzu-hsia learned that his mother had suddenly fallen seriously ill and used the king's carriage to rush to her side. Unfortunately he had not had time to ask for the king's permission and was risking severe punishment. However, when the king learned what Mi had done, he not only did not punish him, but praised his filial piety. Another incident showed the warmth of the affection between the king and his lover: While taking a walk in the king's garden, Mi picked an unusually sweet and delicious peach. Instead of eating the whole peach, Mi ate half and saved the remaining half for the king. King Ling was so touched by Mi's affection for him that he publicly acknowledged Mi's love (Watson, 1964). This story gave rise to the expression "sharing the remaining peach," or "yu-tao," as a term for male homosexuality.

The second incident, recorded in *History of the Former Han*, also involves royalty. Emperor Han Ai-ti (reigned 6 B.C.–A.D. 1) was once in love with the handsome young Dong Xian and was so fascinated by Dong's beauty that he appointed him to a high position in the court. Dong accompanied the Emperor in all his travels and always slept in the same bed. Once, when the two had been taking a nap, the Emperor awoke and saw that the long sleeve of his gown was trapped under the soundly sleeping Dong. He decided to have the sleeve cut off from the gown rather than disturb his lover's sleep (Ban, 1959, Vol. 93). Thus, "the cut sleeve" or "tuan hsiu" became another literary expression for homosexuality.

The third incident was recorded in "The Book of Wei" in Chan-Kuo-Tse (*Intrigues of the Warring States*). During the Warring States period of the Zhou dynasty, a king in the state of Wei had a male companion, Lord Lung-yang. Lung-yang was the king's favorite lover and friend. Once on a fishing trip, after catching about a dozen fish, Lung-yang suddenly burst into tears. When the king asked the reason for this sudden sadness, Lung-yang replied that he was very happy when he caught the first fish until he caught a larger fish. He was thinking of giving away the smaller fish when it struck him that he was in a similar situation. He knew there were persons more beautiful than himself in the world and feared the king might abandon him as he had been prepared to abandon the smaller fish. The king immediately reassured him that this would never happen, and issued an order prohibiting the mention of anyone more beautiful than Lung-yang. People who violated this order would be punished by having their entire families killed (Crump, 1970, p. 440). Lung-yang's name passed into history as another synonym for homosexual love.

The Golden Age of Homosexuality in China

Zhou Dynasty

Ancient Chinese literature is replete with accounts of historical figures who were homosexual, as well as literary expressions of homosexual feeling. One dynastic record even devoted a special section to the emperors' homosexual lovers. A survey of these materials clearly reveals that homosexuality was widely known and often acceptable to ancient China's upper classes. Because only the activities of emperors, princes, high officials, and famous intellectuals were recorded, we do not have direct evidence of how widespread homosexuality was among the common people. However, given the number of homosexual involvements among the upper classes, it is fair to say that ancient China, especially before the Sung dynasty, was the Golden Age of Homosexuality.

The Book of Poetry (*She King*, Shi Jing, or Shih Ching), a collection of poems and folk songs from the early Zhou dynasty (see Chapter 2), contains poems which are the first expression of homosexuality in Chinese literature. What is noteworthy about the poem quoted here is that, just as some heterosexual love poems mention famous female beauties by name, this poem mentions a famous male beauty by name, suggesting that homosexual love was an accepted alternative. The two personal names in the poem, Tsze-too and Tsze-chung, belong to one and the same person, referred to in Chinese histories as the most beautiful gay man of his time.

Shan yew foo-soo
(On the Mountain Is the Mulberry Tree)

On the mountain is the mulberry tree,
In the marsh is the lotus flower.
I do not see Tsze-too,
But I see and like this mad fellow.

On the mountain is the lofty pine,
In the marsh is the spreading water-polygoun.
I do not see Tsze-chung [another name of Tsze-too],
But I see and like this artful boy.

(Legge, 1971)

China's oldest extant historical record of male homosexuality was a passage in *Master Yen's Spring-Autumn Annals*, paraphrased here:

> Qi Jing Kong, the king of Qi State [reigned 547–490 B.C.] was very beautiful, in a feminine fashion. One day, when an officer looked at him lustfully, Qi Jing Kong asked, "Why are you looking at me that way?" The officer replied, "Because you are so very beautiful," and Qi Jing Kong said, "If you have sex with the king, you will receive the death penalty."
>
> Master Yen, the premier, told the king that it was not right to reject sexual desire, and not good to reject love. "The officer's desire for you is not a crime deserving the death penalty."
>
> The king responded by allowing the officer to embrace him as he was bathing. (Author's translation)

At that period of time, it was an act of great courage for an officer to express his desire to have a sexual relationship with his king. Like the poem "Shan yew foo-soo," this tale is clear evidence that in ancient China, homosexuality was tolerated and even accepted.

Other tales from the Spring–Autumn and Warring States periods reflect themes that are characteristic of the royal milieu. Love stories intermingle with details of court intrigue, the jealousy of rivals, and the fear of replacement by new favorites.

One account, for example, tells how homosexual seduction was used as a political and military weapon. Jin Xian Gong, the king of Jin state (reigned 676–651 B.C.) wanted to attack Yu state, but feared Yu's chief military officer, Gong Zhi Qi. Jin's advisor Xun Xi remarked that according to *The History of the Zhou Dynasty*, "a beautiful man can seduce an old man." Therefore Jin Xian Gong sent a beautiful man to Yu State as a spy, ordering him to seduce the king of Yu. Jin's spy succeeded in convincing his royal lover to dismiss Gong Zhi Qi. Gong left the state of Yu, making it an easy conquest for Jin Xian Gong.

Tan, the lover of Chu Xian Wang, the king of Chu state from 369–340 B.C., held a high position and great wealth. The king was enamored of Tan's beauty, but Tan's friend Jiang Yi advised him to protect himself from falling out of favor when he became old and unattractive. On Jiang's advice, Tan told the king that he intended to die with him, and so accompany him forever. The king was so touched that he gave Tan a special title, "Lord An-Ling" (the Lord of An-Ling Area). Frequently, in Chinese homosexual literature, authors mention Lord Lung-yang and Lord An-Ling together.

Shen-hou was a favorite of Chu Wen Wang, king of the state of Chu from 689 to 677 B.C. The king, who loved Shen-hou very deeply, once commented while he was drinking, "You should flee from this country after I die, to avoid being attacked." Shen-hou eventually followed this advice and fled to the state of Zheng, where he again became the king's lover. Eventually Shen-hou's luck ran out: the king's successor had him assassinated for political reasons.

An example of bisexuality is that of Zhao, the homosexual partner of Wei Ling Kong, king of the state of Wei from 534 to 493 B.C. Zhao was also the lover of Wei Ling Kong's mother and of his wife, Nan Tzu. Zhao rebelled against the king and allowed him to leave the country. When the king returned and resumed power, Zhao himself escaped with Nan Tzu. Amazingly, the king and his mother missed Zhao so much that they allowed him and Nan Tzu to return.

Han Dynasty

The Han dynasty ruled China for 400 years and was divided into two periods: the Former Han (Western Han, capital at Changan in the West from 206 B.C. to A.D. 8) and, after an eighteen-year interregnum, the Later Han (Eastern Han, capital at Luoyang in the East from A.D. 25 to 220).

In Western Han there were eleven emperors and one empress (the Queen of Gao-ti, reigned 187–180 B.C.). It is very impressive that ten of the eleven emperors had at least one homosexual lover or expressed some homosexual proclivities (Pan, 1947).

The *History of the (Former) Han Dynasty* (Han Shu) contained a special section describing the emperors' male sexual partners, but the *History of the Later Han Dynasty* (Hou Han Shu) contained no such records. Thus our information about royal homosexuality is restricted to the earlier period. Again, the historical accounts tell us as much about intrigue and jealousy as about love and loyalty.

The founder of the powerful Han dynasty, Guo-ti, reigned from 206 to 195 B.C., and was known by several names, including Gao-ti, Han Gaozu, and Liu Bang. He is considered one of China's greatest emperors. His homosexual relationship with Ji-ru led the great historian Ssuma Chhien (146–86 B.C.) to comment in his *Historical Records* (Shih Chi) that women were not the only people who used their beauty to advantage, and that men, too, often received high positions from emperors or kings by virtue of their sexual attractions. (According to Professor G.D. Pan [1947], the character "ru" in Ji-ru's name means "a man who is like another man's wife.") Besides Ji-ru, Guo-ti took palace eunuchs as lovers.

The account of Wen-ti and Deng Tung has a hint of folklore about it. One can believe that Wen-ti (reigned 179–157 B.C.) was the most parsimonious of the emperors, but can he really have been so thrifty that he refused to throw away old or worn-out clothing? One can also believe that he made an exception in his generosity to his lover Deng Tung, while doubting that he literally gave him a "mountain" of copper for making his own coins. In any case, Deng Tung was known as the richest man of his time, and this was his reward for a loyalty so great that when Wen-ti had a skin abscess he drained it by sucking it. When Wen-ti's son Jing-ti refused to do the same, the emperor reproachfully compared him to Deng Tung. When Jing-ti ascended the throne, he took his revenge on Deng Tung, who eventually died of starvation. (Wen-ti, like Guo-ti, also had relations with some palace eunuchs.)

Wu-ti (156–87 B.C.), known as the Martial Emperor, was an ambitious and brilliant military strategist who expanded his empire into most of the regions included in modern China. It was as a result of Han Wu-ti's expansionist policy that China came into contact with Western culture for the first time. Wu-ti was a bisexual whose male partners included a high official, Han Yen, a court musician, and the great generals Wei Qing and Huo Chu-bin. Thanks to Wu-ti's generosity, Han Yen was reputed to be as wealthy as Deng Tung. It was said that Han Yen's favorite game was tossing away golden balls, and that he lost more than ten daily. Wei Qing, whose sister was also the emperor's lover, was buried in the imperial cemetery.

Some Accounts of Homosexuality from the End of the Han to the Beginning of the Ming Dynasty

Although there are no accounts of homosexuality in *The History of the Later Han Dynasty*, it is clear that the custom continued, because there are records for the period between the Later Han Dynasty and the Three Kingdom period (A.D. 220–280). Perhaps the most interesting is that concerning Liang Ji (A.D. ?–159), who, with his two sisters, ruled for over twenty years. He and his wife actually competed for the love and sexual favors of the servant Chin Gong.

During the Western and Eastern Chin and Southern and Northern Dynasties (A.D. 256–581), male homosexuality seems to have continued to be acceptable in the broader upper-class society (Pan, 1941). A well-known story from the Wei Chin period tells of seven famous scholars, the "Seven Sages of the Bamboo Groves," all of whom had intimate relations with each other. The nineteenth chapter of Liu I Ching's *A New Account of Tales of the World* reports that when two of these scholars were guests in the home of a third, Shan Tao (A.D. 205–283), Shan Tao's wife found them making love (van Gulik, 1961; I. C. Liu, 1976).

This was a historical period of great confusion, as many small states rose and fell, often under the pressure of foreign invasions. There are several accounts of intercultural homosexual relationships and bisexual relationships. There are several accounts (in addition to that of the seven sages) describing affairs among men who, while belonging to the upper classes, did not belong to the royalty or nobility.

One is the account of Xin De-Yuan, a famous scholar living in the Northern Dynasties period (A.D. 386–581). His lover was Pei Rang-zi, an officer of the Norther Qi state and a famous scholar. Another such account describes a relationship that was both homosexual and incestuous, that of Wang Seng-da and Wang Que. Wang Seng-da was a highly placed officer who had an affair with his nephew, Wang Que, a beautiful boy. Wang Seng-da also loved a soldier, Zhu Ling-bao; he released Zhu from the Army, then passed him off as his son to keep him near.

The story of Yu Xin and Xiao Shao suggests that acceptance of homosexuality, while widespread, was not unqualified. Yu Xin (A.D. 513–581) was a famous poet who, when Xiao Shao was young, loved him very much. Later, Xiao Shao gained a high office (the equivalent of governor), and lost his respect for Yu Xin. Yu Xin took his revenge by telling of their past relationship at a banquet, in order to embarrass Xiao Shao.

An especially interesting record is that of Chen Wen-ti and Chen Zi-gao. Chen Wen-ti, also called Chen Chien, was the second emperor of Nan Chen, reigning from A.D. 559–566. Chen Zi-gao, an able general, had a beauty rivaling that of any woman. He dressed in women's clothing and fulfilled the role of queen. What is most interesting about the historical account of their relationship is that it is a rare example of an historical (as opposed to fictional) description of the details of a homosexual relationship. According to this account:

> Chen Chien's penis was very large, so anal intercourse was very painful for Zi-Gao, a mere boy of sixteen. Zi-gao bit down on the bed covers to relieve his pain, biting so hard that the covers were damaged. Chen Chien, not wishing to hurt Zi-gao, stopped and asked, "Have I hurt you?" Zi-gao replied, "My body is yours. I am loved by your love; even death is worthy." By the time Zi-gao had matured fully, his penis was larger than Chen Chien's. (Wuxia, 1909; Author's translation)

Records from the Ming and Ching Dynasties

More historical records are available from the Ming and Ching dynasties (A.D. 1368–1911). From this period we have records of the shiahng gung (different connotations of this term will be explained), giving us a glimpse of homosexuality outside upper-class confines. Also from this period we have the famous *Records of the Cut Sleeve* (Tuan Shiu Pien), the work of an anonymous early nineteenth-century author who compiled approximately fifty famous homosexual case histories (Wuxia, 1909). *Records of the Cut Sleeve* may have been the only book in premodern Chinese literature dealing almost exclusively with male homosexuality. In a modern resource concerning this period, *The Dragon and the Phoenix* (1971), Eric Chou devoted two sections to describing the widespread practice of homosexuality during the Ching dynasty. The first section, "The Manchus Indulge in Homosexuality," described the homosexual relationships of two emperors, Hsien Fong (reigned 1851–1861) and Tung Chih (reigned 1862–1874), with their subordinates. The other section, "The Rabbit Becomes Prime Minister," described how the lover of Emperor Chien Lung (reigned 1736–1795), Ho Shen (1750–1799), became the prime minister as a result of their love relationship. (The word "rabbit" was a slang term for a male homosexual.)

Here we will give two other accounts of famous homosexual relationships occurring during the Ching dynasty. The first concerns the famous and much sought-after Wang Lang. (This is a nickname; Wang is the family name, and "Lang" means simply "young man." His given name was Chi-Chia.) Wang Lang was from Ssu Chou; in his heyday, from the 1640s to 1660s, he was nationally famous for his beauty. When he was thirty years old he went to Chang-an, where he was literally adored by many powerful aristocrats. They were willing to do anything to earn his favors. He was praised by many famous scholars and poets, including Wu Wei-Yeh (1609–1671) and Chien Chien-i (1582–1664) (Hummel, 1942; Pan, 1947).

Another famous homosexual affair was that between the Ching Dynasty's outstanding scholar and official, Pi Yuan, and his lover Li Lang (Hummel, 1942). In 1760, when Pi had passed the highest national examination and earned the title of Chuang-Yuan (top-rated scholar), Li was called "Mrs." Chuang-Yuan. Later, when Pi was a high government official, he surrounded himself with subordinates who shared his orientation. According to the writer Chen Yung, when Pi was the governor of Shensi Province, his mansion was like a homosexual club, always filled with beautiful men who sang, danced, and enjoyed themselves all day long. One day the governor suddenly ordered his chief of staff to bring 500 gunmen and 500 archers to his mansion, explaining that he needed a thousand soldiers to drive out his "rabbits." Doubtless a joke, this remark nonetheless showed how common homosexuality was at the time (Pan, 1947).

At the time this event occurred, the Chien Lung and Chai Ching periods (A.D. 1736–1820), the occupation of "shiahng gung" was a realm of homosexuality outside the upper-class milieu. "Shiahng gung" originally meant "your excellency," "young master of a noble house," or "handsome young man." However, in the Ching dynasty it was also used to refer to male actors who played female roles. Later it was used to refer either to a male actor or to a male homosexual's lover. Thus, shiahng gung came to have a meaning similar to the combined slang terms "drag queen" and "hustler." Later, people came to feel that the term "shiahng gung" was not appropriate; it was changed to "shiahng gu" because "gung" is male and "gu" is female. At this point, "shiahng gung" and "shiahng gu" might have been translated "she-male."

In Beijing, businesses known as "shiahng-gung tang-sze" or "shiahng-gu tang-sze" flourished. The men in the shiahng gung houses dressed, behaved, and spoke like women. They wore perfume and cosmetics, moved like women, and had numerous male admirers. The shiahng gung houses were eventually abolished toward the end of the Ching dynasty and the beginning of the Republic (Pan, 1947).

There are records of another type of outlet for male homosexuals during the Ching dynasty. For example, Nanjing's "Chao Tian Gong" (a Taoist temple) was famous for providing young monks to entertain rich and powerful men for a high fee (*Oriental Daily News*, January 10, 1985). "Chao Tian Gong" has a long history. It was built during A.D. 920–937 and rebuilt in A.D. 1384, but may have functioned as a homosexual brothel only during the Ching dynasty (1644–1911).

Literary Depictions of Male Homosexual Life

The earliest known literary description of homosexual life in China was Pai Hsing-chien's *Poetical Essays on the Supreme Joy* (Thien Ti Yin Tang Ta Lo Fu). Pai Hsing-chien (A.D. 776–826) was the brother of the Tang dynasty's famous poet, Pai chu-yi (A.D. 772–846). Pai Hsing-chien himself was a famous poet and writer. A manuscript of his work was found in the Stone Chamber in Dong-Huang. Since the work was more than a thousand years old, there were many missing parts and unclear passages. The surviving fragments were reproduced in the *Double Plum-Tree Collection* (Yeh, 1914), described in Chapter 3. Generally speaking, the work recorded the historical stories, including those of the shared peach, the cut sleeve, and Lung-yang, as well as recording the homosexual relationships of the Han emperors Gao-ti and Wu-ti. Pai Hsing-chien offered his own conclusion that human sexuality is not limited to heterosexual relationships, and that homosexual intercourse is one expression of human nature.

During the Ming and Ching dynasties, when Chinese classical novels were at their best, many included descriptions of homosexual behavior, some of them surprisingly realistic and detailed, and some even had male homosexuality as their primary or exclusive theme. One of the most famous classical novels, *The Golden Lotus* (Chin Ping Mei) includes homosexual themes. The earliest extant edition of this book was published in 1617, and while there are many subsequent editions, this book relies on a 1957 photocopy of the 1617 edition.

In terms of sexual behavior, the book concentrates on the heterosexual relationships of the main character Hsi-Men Ching with the three women whose names make up the title of the book—Pang Chin-lien (Golden Lotus), Li Ping-erh (Vase), and Chun-mei (Plum Blossom)—and sixteen others. However, the novel also described Hsi-Men's sexual relationships with two men. An example is the following passage from Chapter 34, describing an encounter between Hsi-Men and his young secretary:

> One day, Hsi-Men found his young male servant (age 16) with his face flushed and his lips reddened from drinking. The sight aroused his sexual desire. He took his young servant in his arms, embracing and kissing him. The fragrant tea and cake in the young man's mouth, and the perfume on his body, further aroused Hsi-Men. He pulled up the young servant's garment and stroked his buttocks.... (Author's translation)

The most famous classical Chinese novel was *Dream of the Red Chamber* (Hun-lou Meng), written by Tsao Hsueh-chin (1715?–1763?), and posthumously published in 1792. Though rather reticent in describing sexual behavior, the novel included many descriptions of heterosexual love, and also described some homosexual love affairs in detail. In particular, the homosexual relationships between the main character, Chia Pao-yu, and two other men were touchingly described.

A Mirror of Theatrical Life (Ping-hua Bao Jan), written by Chen Sen in 1849, has been widely recognized as the representative novel about homosexuality (Zhang, 1950). This work expressed strong approval of homosexuality, but did not provide detailed and concrete descriptions of homosexual behavior. The only description of techniques appears in Chapter 23, when the author tells how one character used a water-soaked tree-fungus on the tip of his penis to ease anal penetration and prevent direct contact with his partner's feces during intercourse.

The Ching dynasty novel providing the most detailed and concrete descriptions of homosexual lovemaking would have to be *Pleasant Spring and Fragrant Character* (Yi-chun Xiang-zhi). This novel, written under the pseudonym Xin Yue Zhu Ren, was so rare it was not even included in standard bibliographies listing works with sexual themes (e.g., Sun Kai-ti, 1982; Liu Cun-ren, 1982). However, it was included on lists of books officially banned during the Dao Guang (1821–1850) and Tung Chih (1862–1874) periods. As a banned book, it was rarely circulated, and the edition referred to here is a handwritten copy stored in the Beijing Library. The novel appears to have been written between 1796 and 1843, and can safely be said to belong to the first half of the nineteenth century.

The work contains four volumes, respectively titled *Wind*, *Flower*, *Snow*, and *Moon*. Each volume is an independent story with five chapters and contains numerous descriptions of homosexual behavior and acts. One of the simpler, more easily understood portions, quoted here, illustrates the wealth of detail contained in this novel. The scene takes place in Chapter 1, Volume 1, between Li Zun-xian, an eighteen-year-old student, and Sun Yi-zhi, a thirteen-year-old student:

> Li's penis had reached Sun's anus and was fully erect but could not enter. Despite several attempts in different ways, Li still could not succeed in entering Sun. Meanwhile Sun was screaming with pain and begged Li to stop. Li told Sun that he did not want to hurt him, but the really wonderful sensations would come later. Li also told Sun that it would help if Sun moved his buttocks. Sun replied that it hurt everywhere, so Li might as well come into him.
>
> Li instructed Sun to hold his own buttocks and then bear down. He would enter Sun at that time. Meanwhile, Li lubricated his penis with his saliva, and with a strong push succeeded in entering Sun. Sun's inside was still quite tight and dry. Li used another strong push, inserting the whole length of his penis. Li then forcefully pushed up and down, in and out. Gradually, Sun's inside began to feel smooth and slippery. Li could now enter and withdraw easily. Sun began to feel as if liquid were flooding his inside, and had a strong sensual feeling. He began to move his buttocks up and down until he could hardly breathe and indulged himself in this pleasure.
>
> Li knew then that Sun was enjoying himself, and pushed his penis with great force while Sun was resting, catching his breath. It was at this point that Sun reached his sexual climax. He moaned, "Dear brother!" and turned around and kissed Li on the mouth. (Translated by Ruan & Tsai, 1987)

Descriptions of homosexuality also appeared in the famous short stories of the Ming period. For example, such descriptions appeared in *Stories for Enlightened Men* (Yu-Shih Ming-Yen), *Stories to Warn Men* (Ching-Shih Dong-Yen), and *Stories to Awaken Men* (Hsin-Shih Heng-Yen), collections edited by Feng Meng-lung (A.D. 1574–1646); and in *Amazing Stories* (Pa-An Ching-Chi) and *Second Series of Amazing Stories* (Erh-Kuo Pa-an Ching-chi), collections edited by Ling Meng-chu (A.D. 1580–1644).

For example, in Volume 10 of *Stories to Awaken Men,* there is a description of an encounter between an old transvestite and the young San Mao:

> San Mao was a beautiful boy. One day while taking shelter from the rain in a temple, he encountered an "old lady" with whom he engaged in sexual relations. It was only after the sodomy that he realized the "old lady," was actually a man of 47 years. (Translated by Ruan & Tsai, 1987)

An example from Volume 26 of *Amazing Stories* is the portrayal of a homosexual love affair between an older monk, Ta-chueh, and the young monk Chih-yan. The story was set in Sichuan province, in a temple called "Tai Ping" which had ten monks. One of them, Chih-yan, was a very handsome, attractive, and seductive young man. His master was the old monk Ta-chueh, a bisexual who was very lustful. The older monk who, though approaching fifty, was as virile as a young man, summoned the young monk to his bed nightly. Their erotic passion was said to be beyond description (Ling, 1982).

Varying Perspectives on Homosexuality

While these excerpts show that homosexuality was recognized and often accepted, more extreme attitudes were also expressed. Some of the traditional Chinese literature glorified homosexuality and some condemned it. The best example of the first approach was *The Mirror of Theatrical Life,* previously mentioned as the most representative novel of homosexuality. Some speculate that the book's main character, Tien Chun-hang, actually represents the famous Ching scholar-bureaucrat, Pi yuan. (Some elaborate Chinese puns on the two names are involved.) It is clear that this character expresses the views of the author, Chen Sen, when he eloquently praises the charms of catamites:

> Across tens of thousands of miles, through five thousand years of history, nothing and nobody is better than a catamite. Those who do not love a catamite should not be taken seriously. Elegant flowers, beautiful women, the shining moon, rare books, and grand paintings, all those supreme beauties are appreciated by everyone. However, these beauties often are not in one place. Catamites are different. They are like elegant flowers and not grass or trees; they are like beautiful women who do not need make-up; they are like a shining moon or tender cloud, yet they can be touched and played with; they are like rare books and grand paintings, and yet they can talk and converse; they are beautiful and playful and yet they also are full of change and surprise. The loss of a catamite cannot be compensated

by any beauty in history. The gain of a catamite makes the loss of a historic beauty a small matter. I do not comprehend why it is supposed to be normal for a man to love a woman, but abnormal for a man to love a man. Passion is passion whether to a man or a woman. To love a woman but not a man is lust and not passion. To lust is to forget passion. If one treasures passion he would not be lewd. (Translated by Ruan & Tsai, 1987)

Later, Tien Chun-hang utters more extravagant praise of catamites:

A catamite is an ultimate friend of beauty and virtue: His look is tender, elegant and beautiful; his skin is snow-white and his body is soft yet firm; his appearance is charming and lovely; his manner is seductive and enchanting; his affection is innocent and shy; his adornment is grand and splendid. Add to all these extraordinary qualities, music and dance, and elegant surroundings, and one experiences something like exaltation. Such then is a pleasure, a person.... (Translated by Ruan & Tsai, 1987)

Tien's celebration of homosexual love hints at another social reality. His plaintive remark, "I do not comprehend why it is supposed to be normal for a man to love a woman, but abnormal for a man to love a man," was addressed to those contemporaries who considered homosexuality a deviant behavior. Though not extensively or severely punished, this life-style did receive its share of condemnation.

Concern about such condemnation certainly influenced some authors. For example, the Ming dynasty author Zhang Jun-ying wrote a book entitled *The Classic of the Human Mirror* (Ren Jing Jing), published in 1641, in which he explicitly portrayed homosexual behavior. However, he made a point of declaring that the "mirror" of his book's title reflected both virtue and evil, and he implied that homosexuality was the evil his "mirror" was intended to reflect. Even *Pleasant Spring and Fragrant Character*, with its explicit descriptions of homosexual behavior, implicitly condemned homosexuality. The cruelty of the punishment inflicted upon one of the novel's homosexual characters is incomparable. In Book 2, the main homosexual character, Shan Siu-yen, was portrayed as very beautiful. Many men sought after him, risking their fortunes and remaining unmarried to earn his love. Yet the manner of Shan's eventual demise was horrifying:

...an object like a fish-hook was forced into his [Shan's] anus and pulled out his intestines slowly and repeatedly until his death.... (Translated by Ruan & Tsai, 1987)

The inclusion of this incident may have been the author's way of avoiding punishment for his detailed descriptions of homosexual behavior. It also reflected the social reaction to homosexuality during the last thousand years. Such stories were in marked contrast with the positive images of homosexuality in the ancient literature.

In addition to varying evaluations of homosexuality, there were two interpretations of its basis to be found in traditional Chinese literature—the "nature" and "nurture" theories familiar to Westerners. The first interpretation attributes homosexuality to natural endowment. For example, the famous Ching author, Yuan Mei (A.D. 1716–1797), in Sui-Yuan Shi Hua (*Critical Reviews in Poems at the Garden Shi*), described a man who looked like a woman and could not get along with his wife. He was portrayed as loving to play and sleep with men and feeling that he would rather be a handsome man's concubine than a beautiful woman's husband. He would say to himself that human beings are born with different characters just as trees grow different kinds of branches (Pan, 1947). Thus, in this author's view, one is "born homosexual."

The second interpretation attributed homosexuality to nurture, that is, environmental causes. For example, Chi Yun (1724–1805), in his *Notes of the Yueh-Wei Heritage* (1800), stated that lust for a woman was a result of a natural sexual drive, but not lust for a catamite. He claimed that such desires resulted from learning during childhood, or seduction by rich, powerful, and deviant people (Pan, 1947).

Little, if any, evidence was available for either view. No systematic or scientific studies of the basis of homosexuality have been made either in traditional Chinese society or in today's China.

The Dark Age of Homosexuality in Modern China

Considering the many and varied records of homosexuality in ancient China, one would expect to find evidence of homosexuality in modern China. However, literature regarding contemporary homosexuality is scarce at best. Thus, for example, in Weinberg and Bell's 550-page book on homosexuality, *Homosexuality: An Annotated Bibliography* (1972), not a single study or record of homosexuality in China is listed. Parker's three-volume bibliography on homosexuality (1971, 1977, and 1985) includes 9,924 items, but only two articles, both from gay publications, on Chinese homosexuality.

This scarcity of literature on Chinese homosexuality is at least partially due to the prohibitions against homosexuality, which are especially strong in contemporary China. Gay men are frequently punished and understandably reluctant to reveal their identities. As a result, it is extremely difficult to obtain any realistic and objective information on gay life in China.

These problems are exacerbated by the fact that, since the regime's inception in 1949, objective information on homosexuality has been almost completely unavailable in the People's Republic of China. The changes and improvements in gay rights which have occurred in other parts of the world in the past twenty years or so, and information about gay life outside China, are rarely reported inside China. The few reports on gay life in the outside world have primarily been used as examples of the "decline and evil of Western civilization." These circumstances create a sense of isolation among Chinese gays which is clearly evident in their remarks below, and which adds to the difficulties in learning about their situation.

Thus it was a genuine breakthrough when, through a rather unique and unexpected set of events which will be described, the author obtained 56 letters from gay individuals in China in 1985 and 1986. In these letters were descriptions of the personal lives, problems, and aspirations of the writers. Though these informants are not a random and representative sample, they come from all walks of life, and all regions of China, and the information they provided appears to be the first and only such material on contemporary Chinese gay life to have been obtained by any scholar. Only in the last few years have a few enterprising journalists succeeded in gleaning some information about gay life. What they learned will be described in the section titled "Social Status of Homosexuals in Mainland China," and generally confirms the information in the 56 letters received by the author. A sociological analysis of these letters should fill in some of the void on contemporary Chinese gay life.

In 1985, the author, using the pen name Jin-ma Hua, published an article titled "Homosexuality: An Unsolved Puzzle" in a widely circulated health magazine, *To Your Good Health* (Ruan, 1985a). The article pointed out that homosexuality has occurred in all nations, all social strata, and in all eras in human history. It acknowledged that in some countries, in some historical periods, homosexuals were severely punished and sometimes even received the death penalty, adding that such persecution was perhaps an example of how majorities subjugate minorities in human societies. The article went on to assert that homosexuals should not be persecuted for failing to reproduce; that the number of homosexuals in any society is substantial and greater than laypeople realize; that homosexuals' problems should not be ignored and that they deserve a reasonable social status; and that homosexuals do not differ from heterosexuals in such qualities as intelligence, physical strength, and creativity or the ability to maintain stable relationships.

The publication of this article attracted considerable attention. Many letters, most from gay men, were written to the magazine's editor in response to the article. Then, five months after its first publication, the bulk of the article was reprinted in the most popular and widely read magazine in China, *The (Chinese) Reader's Digest*. By April 1986, a total of 60 letters had been received by the editor of *To Your Good Health* and forwarded to the author. (Both articles will be referred to below as "Hua's article.")

Considering the strength of the legal, moral, and social prohibitions against homosexuality, this apparently small number of responses is in fact quite substantial. Forty-three of the letter-writers revealed their identities. Names, geographic locations, and occupations were given. It was a general sentiment that the magazines' editors and the article's author had earned the trust of these men. Thus one man wrote that "If the magazine and the author are courageous enough and willing to risk the consequences...speaking for homosexuals in a fair and objective manner...they would not doublecross us" (Letter 52).

All 60 letters were written by men; other materials had to be used for the section on lesbianism, and heterosexual women's attitudes toward homosexuality remain unexplored. Fifty-six letters were from gay men, who all approved of the article and thanked its author. Of the remaining four letters, two disapproved of the article's editorial position; the third suggested a way to convert gays to heterosexuality; and the last was written by a transsexual.

In this section, we will discuss the expressions of approval and disapproval contained in the letters. The next section will consist of a thorough content analysis. To preserve the anonymity of the people who wrote the letters, each one will be referred to by a number.

Approval and Disapproval Expressed in Responses to "A Defense of Homosexual Rights"

The following excerpts are representative of the manner of expression in the letters received and the kinds of reasoning used to justify their authors' viewpoints. A striking aspect of the letters from gay men is their immense relief at having an opportunity to express their feelings.

> Hua's article on homosexuality provides me with a soothing sense of relief never before experienced in my life. It also gives me hope about my life and my future.... (Letter 11)
> I am extremely grateful for Hua's objective, humane, scientific and fair critique on homosexuality. (Letter 24)

The publication of this article is a great event in the medical field. It is a salvation of thought, a fruit of progressive advancement. To homosexuals, it is true "good news." We admire your courage and scientific attitude toward this matter. (Letter 25)

This article is truly great. It gives us, a small number of homosexuals, a spiritual uplift. It gives me the second life and takes me to the spring of my life. (Letter 28, written by a college student who had attempted suicide)

Of the two letters expressing disapproval of homosexuality, one (Letter 57) came from a medical college in the northwest region of China, and the other (Letter 58) came from a teacher in a factory training center in the northeastern region of China.

Hua's article is attempting to legitimize homosexual life and is not an objective treatment of the subject matter. (Letters 57 and 58)

Homosexuality is an evil product of capitalistic society. Homosexuality brings with it bad influence on our socialist society. It is our obligation to point out our view in stopping this product of spiritual pollution. (Letter 57)

In a tone reminiscent of the Cultural Revolution, the writer of Letter 58 added:

We should absolutely prohibit homosexuality.... Widespread homosexuality will lead to epidemic deterioration of our racial spirit and destroy our society.... The reason that people despise, prohibit, punish and persecute homosexuals is precisely that the behavior is evil, ugly, opposed to human morality, and an insult to human dignity, promotes crime among youth, ruins their mental and physical health, leads to the destruction of our race and civilization.... It is imperative that we expose homosexuality lest it create a flood that sweeps away our marital, moral, legal and customary dam and destroys our socialist civilization. (Letter 58)

An Analysis of Self-Descriptions of Male Homosexuals in China

The primary goal here is to provide a collective portrait based on these letters. It is hoped that an analysis will provide some initial insight into gay life in contemporary China. It is not claimed that the writers of the letters are a representative sample of China's gay population, but it is reasonable to assume that many of their feelings and experiences represent the reality of broad segments of that population. For ease of presentation, the results of the content analysis of these letters are grouped under several headings.

Demographic Analysis

Of the 56 letters from gay men, 34 indicated the writer's age. Three were 20 years or younger, 25 were between 21 and 30 years old, 3 between 31 and 40, 2 between 41 and 50, and 1 between 51 and 60 years old. It is obvious from the foregoing that the majority were in their 20s. Although the same is true of the population in general, the concentration in the 21–30 age bracket is not necessarily representative; it may mean that, for some reason, members of this group felt freer to express themselves.

Forty-six writers indicated their geographic locations. The greatest number came from Shanghai, China's most populous city. However, it is important to note that letters came from almost every region of the country.

Judging from their writing styles, it appears that all the letter writers had at least some high school education. Eleven clearly indicated that they either were attending or had graduated from college, one was pursuing a master's degree, and one a doctoral degree. Among the occupations listed were college professor, instructor, high school teacher, actor, soldier, factory worker, government bureaucrat, and high school, college, or graduate student.

Gay Life and Its Problems

Many letters expressed their writers' conflicting desires for confidentiality and a chance to overcome their isolation. Many explicitly requested protection of their confidentiality, often in strikingly similar language. The writer of Letter 19 said, "Please keep this in utmost secret. I would not know how to face others if my identity is known"; and the writer of Letter 24 said, "If this is known by the public my future would be ruined." Yet twenty requested the names and addresses of other gay people in the apparent hope that either the magazine or the article's author could facilitate a gay network.

Twenty-two letters mentioned marital status. Twelve writers were not married; eight were currently married, including six with children; and two had been divorced. All those who were currently married said that they had married in response to family and social pressures. They were not sexually interested in their wives and seldom engaged in sexual relations with them. All said they continue to have a strong homosexual orientation, but do not feel that they have any choice but to live a lie. Their wives have absolutely no knowledge of their sexuality. They feel extremely guilty about their inability to truly love and give love to their wives. They constantly suffer tremendous pain because of the necessity of living a double life and resent what they see as their own hypocrisy. For example, Letter 1 said:

> I am a 29-year-old young man.... I am not interested in the female sex at all. I do not even want to have any physical contact with them. However, among the men that I have encountered, some would occupy my body and soul.... I am particularly interested in one man and my love for him is beyond description. He is a little smaller than I am, but I fall for him in every respect I can think of. This feeling deepens every day. It has been ten years but my feeling for him has not been changed. Of course I wish I could live with him, be with him—even just sitting quietly with him, I would be very happy. Of course I wish to have a sexual relationship with him but my mind stops and controls me from doing this. I regard him as my spiritual supporter. I obtain my spiritual satisfaction through him. Frequently when I thought of him I would masturbate to fulfill my sexual desire. This strong, persistent, monogamous and inner-directed, everlastingly devoted feeling toward him has continued for over 10 years and is unmatched even among normal heterosexual relationships.... During the last 10 years or so, my life had an interesting twist. When I was 25 years old, a woman fell deeply in love with me. I could not tell her about my true feelings. She insisted on marrying me no matter what. I could not do anything to discourage her. Finally I gave in and married her. I was living in a completely different world. I seldom had sexual relations with her. But on one of those very rare occasions I impregnated her. She knows nothing about my deep secret. This relationship has created pain in my heart and my life. I have been in love and devoted my love to him all this time. I think my love for him will never change for the rest of my life. However, the love is a deep secret. He would not understand nor would he be aware of this. My heart is full of contradiction and pain. I pretend to be happy in front of others, but when alone I cry with pain.

Those who are not married seem to suffer just as deeply for they, too, are lonely:

> The pain that homosexuals suffer most lies not in homosexuality, but in their inability to find suitable lovers. All homosexuals lock their feelings in their hearts. They are so afraid of being discovered that it makes it impossible to live their lives. (Letter 10)
> In this vast world where can I find that 5% to 10% true in heart? (Letter 47)

> I am longing to love others (homosexuals) and to be loved. I
> have met some other homosexuals but I have doubts about this type
> of love. With all the pressure I was afraid to reveal myself and ruined
> everything. As a result, we departed without showing each other
> homosexual love. As I am growing older my homosexual desire in-
> creases. This is too troublesome and too depressing for anyone. I
> thought about death many times. When you are young you cannot
> fall in love and when you are old you will be alone. Thinking of this
> makes the future absolutely hopeless. (Letter 8)

Clearly, the chief source of pain for China's gay men derives from
the fear of societal punishment, including arrest, and possible sentence to labor reform camp or prison. The mental pressure and anguish
arising from the fear that their true identity will be discovered is often
unbearable.

Those who were serving prison terms for their homosexuality at the
time Hua's article appeared could not possibly have read it, much less
responded to it. However, Letter 22 described the testimony of one man
who had been imprisoned. This man was an excellent physics teacher
and had been the director of academic affairs in a high school. His homosexual relationships were voluntary and had been initiated by others.
He was arrested in September 1983 and sentenced to a five-year prison
term for his homosexual acts. Since the publication of Hua's article, this
man's colleagues, friends, and relatives were reported to have changed
their negative attitudes toward him. His superior actually visited him in
prison, but his sentence remained unaltered.

The social pressure, pain, and inner conflict homosexuals suffer can
be so intense that they come to consider or even attempt suicide. Of the
56 who responded to Hua's article, 15, or more than 25%, mentioned
suicide attempts. One such story follows:

> I am an agriculture college student. I will be graduating this
> year. In 1981 I fell in love with a senior student. I was only 17 then
> and had no understanding at all about homosexuality. The mental
> anguish was so unbearable that I was eventually diagnosed as having
> a "reactive psychosis." I took a year's "leave of absence." In 1983,
> still quite confused about homosexuality, I mistakenly overdosed my-
> self with sleeping pills and was hospitalized for four days before
> getting out of danger. (Letter 28)

Aspirations

Of all the hopes and dreams expressed in these moving letters, three
types of aspirations were outstanding. The first concerned the human
rights issue—the belief that society should accept homosexuals and their

right to express their sexuality without social or legal condemnation. The second concerned the issue of freedom to interact with other homosexuals—the wish that society would provide them with means to make contacts and form relationships, just as it does for heterosexuals. The third concerned the issue of knowledge—the wish that objective and scientific studies would be conducted and publicized in order to improve societal understanding.

The following excerpts are typical of the 17 letters advocating protection of homosexual rights:

> There should be open discussion about the issue (of homosexual rights) and homosexuals should be given legal status. (Letter 10)
>
> Homosexual sex is one form of sexual behavior. Because of the problem of population explosion we are facing today, homosexual sex is one effective means of population control. Why do we insist on having a homosexual man marry a woman? Without love, marriage is a mere reproductive machine. Mentally one suffers from the constant disharmony of family life. Physically, one is constantly confronted with the unpleasant experience of contradiction. Without a homosexual companion, how can one have motivation for his career? Homosexuals should be granted the same right as heterosexuals to fulfill their sexual needs. We are a very populous nation; we need to improve homosexuals' status and be concerned with their problems and pains. (Letter 32)

In 20 letters, the hope that some agency would facilitate social contacts among homosexuals took the form of a request that "Dr. Hua" or his publishers do so. In Hua's article, two actual cases of gay life in Hubei and Shanghai had been described. All 20 letters requested the names and addresses of these two men in order to establish contact with them. The tone of some requests, as in Letter 43, was very earnest and urgent.

> The greatest pain for us, the homosexuals, is our inability to express our deepest inner sorrow. We have to hide our feelings in front of others. I therefore beg you to fulfill my wish by giving me the names and addresses of other homosexuals. This may help me find the will to go on living. The pain in my heart makes me extremely despairing. (Letter 43)
>
> I hope to contact other homosexuals through your magazine in order to work out ways to deal with our future. (Letter 10)
>
> I hope you can become homosexuals' go-between and provide a bridge for the great many homosexuals (to contact one another) and bring them hope and happiness. (Letter 25)

Some men, though they did not use the word for "club," expressed the wish to create this type of organization. For example:

I fantasized that there would be a place where homosexuals can converse and interact freely. I fantasized having a lover. But fantasy is not real. In reality, homosexuals do not automatically love all other homosexuals. They choose their partners just like heterosexuals. But where can I find them? In this wide world all homosexuals hide their true identity. It is so much more difficult for a homosexual to find his ideal partner than a heterosexual. I sometimes was tempted to openly seek a homosexual friend. But how can I? I do not think a homosexual person will do any harm to the country and other people. But why can't we openly discuss homosexuality? We should provide ways for exclusive homosexuals to contact one another. I sincerely wish that our country and related governmental agencies could openly show their concern about our problems. (Letter 8)

There were 18 letters pointing out the need for development and/or publication of more information about homosexuality. The following excerpt is representative of these concerns:

A special column should be established to discuss the homosexual problems in comprehensive and in-depth fashion in order for society, especially the public security, judicial departments, party and governmental propaganda organizations, to have an accurate perspective and provide a more reasonable treatment of the homosexuals....

I hope you (the magazine) could invite famous sociologists, doctors, even homosexuals as a team to do an in-depth study on the extent and current condition of homosexuals in our country and to find reasonable ways to deal with them. If you want my humble service on this I would be more than happy to do my best. (Letter 25)

Four of the letters mentioned "underground" (not open or approved) studies then being made of homosexuals in China. One 24-year-old indicated that he had helped a 60-year-old university professor in Beijing, who had himself been gay for decades, to collect data on homosexuals. As part of his work he had traveled to 18 different cities and provinces throughout China. He had found homosexuals everywhere he went. He reported:

Among those places, Beijing, Shanghai, Guangzhow, Wuhan, Nanjing, Shenyang, Fuzhou, and Changsa were most notable (in having a large number of homosexuals). Among those (homosexuals), intellectuals seemed the most numerous. Others include workers, public security officers, etc. It appeared that the number had increased substantially in the last few years...many of those were unfamiliar faces. (Letter 26)

Sadly, 21 men asked how they might be "healed." Apparently they felt that a conversion to heterosexuality might be the only way to resolve their dilemma.

Sexual Psychology and Sexual Behavior

There were very few concrete discussions of sexual behavior, but some men did relate some of their personal experiences.

> I am a genuine male. I am 27 years old. I have been seeking homosexual love for many years. I have not experienced heterosexual love and am not interested in it at all. When I saw some healthy bearded men (I myself am bearded), my member would automatically erect. I was always tempted to touch others' penises in a crowded bus, in a dark movie theater, a bath house... but my rationality stopped me.... In those lonely and sleepless nights I wish I had a strong man lying right next to me. (Letter 27)

> I am a 16-year-old high school student with a masculine appearance. I am not into girls at all. However, I am very moved by males, especially the handsome and strong ones. When I talked with one of them I was so happy. When I was with someone I liked I would be elated. I would snuggle up to him. When I saw an attractive man in a movie, on television or even in a magazine I would experience the excitement of the pre-ejaculation state. (Letter 36)

> I am 26 years old. I have been married for two years and have a child. But I only like muscular, well-built men. I love to see their well-built naked bodies. The more I see them the more excited I get. Sometimes I reach an orgasmic state and ejaculate. This orgasmic feeling was quite clear and was much better than with my wife. My wife is very tender to me. She often rubs my body very softly while we are in bed and sometimes until I fall asleep. She cannot arouse my sexual interest in her. During sexual intercourse with my wife I sometimes get an erection by thinking of some beautiful young man I've met, but frequently I have to stop halfway. (Letter 54)

> I am a 29-year-old man. When I was 15 I was a very nice-looking man. Many people liked me. There was a 17-year-old man I met. We fell in love. We kissed, embraced, and finally we had sex. I played the woman's role. We met everyday and frequently had sex. I felt great and ejaculated myself. (Letter 1)

One man from Shichuan province, who said his nicknames were "cute little fellow" and, sometimes, "buttocks queen," shared what he knew about homosexual hygiene. He felt that with proper hygienic methods, homosexual sex was safe. He told of his own feelings in the following manner:

I am a male homosexual. I like the well-built and deeply tanned young men with large members. When I saw them I felt like they had already entered me. I felt extremely elated and eventually erected and ejaculated. I have had anal sex with more than 200 men, my buttocks have been entered more than 1,000 times. (Letter 32)

Some letters expressed discomfort with or dislike of women. For example, a man from Hunan province said:

I was forced to marry a woman partially because of the obligation to have a child and partially to stop the gossip. I have a child but I have been seeking homosexuals for more than 20 years. I feel great distaste for some women's bad behavior, such as irrationality, gossiping, cursing, dependency, and so on. I dislike having sex with women. (Letter 41)

Another man, a resident of Beijing, said:

I first felt homosexual desire when I was 16. I have had several homosexual encounters. In 1984 I got married. I thought this marriage would gradually change my sexuality, but that did not happen. I seldom initiate sexual relations with my wife; if and when I do it is to comfort her. In reality, I resent any part of a woman's body (including breasts). Their (women's) body shape and muscles are not as beautiful as men's. It has been more than a year (since I got married) and I have yet to feel anything while having sex with a woman. (Letter 35)

Social Status of Homosexuals in Mainland China

The social situation of homosexuals is subject to an extreme expression of the same ambiguity and arbitrariness that characterize government policy and social attitudes toward other sexual behaviors. The lack of public discussion concerning homosexuality makes it extremely difficult for Westerners to gain a clear picture of the social status of homosexuals. Thus Norrgard (1990) eventually had to take her search for Chinese lesbians to Hong Kong (see below). The first impression Westerners receive is one of deceptive calm. Thus Kristof (1990) writes:

Homosexuality is rarely discussed in China's press or in routine conversations. Most Chinese assert that they have never known a homosexual and that there must be extremely few in Chinese society. In large cities, particularly in the southern city of Canton, homosexuals meet in certain bars or parks. They sometimes refer to each other in the Cantonese dialect as geilo, or gay guy. There are no advocacy groups for homosexuals in China. But if the nation lacks an outspoken gay community, it also lacks the invective and bitter hostility that is sometimes directed toward homosexuals in the West. There are no common insults in Chinese related to sexual orientation. Most Chinese frown on homosexuality, but characterize it as improper or in poor taste rather than a sin. The police generally are oblivious to signals of homosexuality, in part because it is common for Chinese of the same sex to hold hands as a sign of friendship. But, homosexuals are occasionally arrested and sentenced to brief jail terms. (Kristof, 1990)

In fact, although there is no specific statement concerning the status of homosexuals in the current Criminal Law of the People's Republic of China, Article 106 says, "All hooliganism should be subjected to arrest and sentence." In practice, homosexual activity has been included in "hooliganism." As noted, even the small sample of letters the author received contained a report of a man who had received a five-year jail term for homosexuality, and additional examples will be given.

Silence, especially a silence based on repression and enforced ignorance, must not be mistaken for approval or tolerance. When public figures do speak out on homosexuality, it is usually to condemn it. For example, one of the most famous attorneys in China today, Mr. Dun Li, when asked to express his opinion concerning homosexuality, said:

Homosexuality, though it exists in different societies and cultures, with some minor exceptions is considered abnormal and disdained. It disrupts social order, invades personal privacy and rights and leads to criminal behavior. As a result, homosexuals are more likely to be penalized administratively and criminally. (Ruan, 1985)

In 1987, a leading forensic psychiatrist, Dr. Zheng Zhanbei, expressed himself in similar terms, asserting that homosexuality is against social morality, interferes with social security, damages the physical and mental health of adolescents, and ought to be a crime (Wan, 1988).

Another common reaction to the suggestion that homosexuality exists in China is denial. This is the stance of Mr. Z. Liu, a well-known newspaper reporter and editor of a famous magazine, who is quite familiar with the approach of Chinese authorities toward special problems. After two years of study in Chicago, Liu described his American experience in *Two Years in the Melting Pot* (1984). By his own account, his exposure to a more liberal view of homosexuality had little effect on his attitudes:

One group on campus, calling itself the gay and lesbian Illini, met every week. I was enormously curious about this group, which concerned itself with issues of homosexuality, but I never ventured to go to any of their meetings. I inquired of friends, however, to find out who these people were and what they did. One of my friends argued that love between those of the same sex is natural and has existed throughout history—during the Roman Empire, it was even made legal, he said. I disagreed, saying that it wouldn't be good for society to open up this issue. In old China, homosexuality was practiced by a few rich people, but the general public didn't approve.

Yet another reaction is to admit that perhaps homosexuality does exist in China, but to insist that when it occurs it is the result of Western influence. This was what was meant when, in rigid ideological fashion, Letter 57 referred to "spiritual pollution." A formal expression of this view appeared in an official newspaper, the *Beijing Daily News*, which identified homosexuality as one of the "Western social diseases," originating in "Western ideology and thoughts" (press release by United Press International, February 4, 1987).

Finally, there are those who, when faced with undeniable evidence of homosexuality, respond by seeking to eliminate it. Thus Wan Ruixiong, a writer who, after spending considerable time conducting interviews, wrote a lengthy report on homosexuality in China, concluded that homosexuality is a crime and expressed the hope that it will someday be abolished (Wan, 1988).

Even most Chinese physicians still fail to recognize homosexuality as simply one possible sexual orientation. In Harbin, one of the largest cities in northeastern China, physicians still use the discredited approach of "treating" homosexuality with aversive techniques. According to one report:

> When homosexuals are treated for what most Chinese doctors regard as their mental illness, they are sometimes given painful electric shocks to discourage erotic thoughts. An alternative approach is to offer herbal medicines that induce vomiting. In either case, the idea is to stimulate an extremely unpleasant reaction that will be associated thereafter with erotic thoughts and thus reduce the patients' ardor. Both approaches... are hailed by doctors in China as remarkably successful in "curing" homosexuality. (Kristof, 1990)

The people subjected to this treatment had not had any criminal charges brought against them, but were sent by family members who were upset by their homosexuality.

It is obvious that the fears of condemnation expressed by the men who responded to Hua's article were entirely realistic. And it is not at all surprising that Hui Fu, a Hong Kong journalist, who spent 10 months traveling China in search of information on gays, found that most were closeted and the few who were not were extremely cautious. He commented, "It was not really easy for me to find them [gays] or penetrate into their circle" (see Ruan & Chong, 1987).

Nevertheless, in the course of his visits to nearly 25 major cities, Fu did manage to make contact with homosexuals and other sexual minorities and interview them about their lifestyles. His account of what he learned was eventually published in a Taiwanese weekly magazine, and it is summarized here.

Not only are most Chinese gays closeted, but those who are active in their lifestyle can only meet in a limited number of places, such as public restrooms, parks, shopping centers, and public baths. For example, one man said that there are certain public restrooms in Beijing that many homosexuals frequently bicycle to in order to meet each other and engage in sexual activity. Other favorite meeting spots are scattered throughout the city's busiest sections, including two shopping centers and the famous Tienanmen Square and Ritan Park. Everyday, after 6:00 P.M., many gays converge on these places. The gays Fu met there included men from every walk of life: factory workers, farmers, students, intellectuals, soldiers, athletes, entertainers, and even policemen.

In Shanghai, the favorite after-dark gathering spot was in front of the Central Post Office. The men who gathered there were very fashion-conscious, and hair lotion, perfume, shirts with high pointed collars, and tight pants were particularly in style. Men strutted back and forth on the street, gesturing as if they were waiting for someone.

Fu was sure he would find gay men in Sian, an ancient walled city and former capital of China which has enjoyed many thousands of years of tradition and culture. Yet he found no one during his two-day stay until just before his departure, when he went into a public restroom located near the city wall. There he met several gay men. One of them, a retired soldier, described his experiences in detail.

The soldier said he had been married, but that his love life had changed four years earlier when he encountered several gay men engaging in oral sex in a public restroom. From that day on, he continued to visit there nearly every night. Other gay men in Sian have also come out of the closet, but, for fear of legal consequences, they are mostly found in secluded places such as public restrooms or the park. Anyone who is caught in a homosexual act is automatically found guilty, subject to immediate arrest and a mandatory jail sentence. The retired soldier said that he personally had witnessed such a case when two men were apprehended as they came out of a public restroom together. One of them was arrested on the spot and given a nine-year prison term after a summary trial.

Fu found that Lanchow, a city of two million people located in northwestern China, is known as an oasis in the desert. Yet the "oasis" consists of only two public restrooms where gays can meet. A 20-year-old man told Fu that there are more than 100 known gays in the city, but they can only meet at the restrooms of the Workers' Cultural Center and the People's Political Consultative Conference building. Fu also discovered an unlighted public restroom in a narrow dead-end alley where, he said, many gay people congregate after dark.

The official denial of a significant gay presence in China clearly contradicts reality. This entire viewpoint is fabricated of misconceptions. Homosexuality is not restricted to a few rich and powerful men; it is found in all walks of life and among all age groups. It is not a Western import; many illustrious figures in China's long history were homosexual. Besides, most of the men who wrote in response to Hua's article had been born after the 1949 revolution and grew up in an era of isolation; several came from remote regions. They are clearly native products.

Current unrealistic policies contribute to a number of problems. Today in mainland China there is an acute housing shortage. Since there are virtually no private rooms for anyone in the family home, many homosexuals are forced to meet elsewhere. Public restrooms are one of the few available locations for social and sexual liaisons. In these unsanitary conditions, gay men are forced to increase their risk of contracting and spreading contagious diseases—including sexually transmitted diseases—perhaps increasing their vulnerability to AIDS. Moreover, in a country in which all medical care is provided under the auspices of a government which denies their basic human rights, those who do contract AIDS or other STDs can hardly be expected to seek treatment or even to discuss their problems in private.

It is time—past time—for the Chinese government to change its policies. Not only must it recognize the rights of gay people and develop educational programs promoting public acceptance of their lifestyle, it must begin promoting safe sex practices, ultimately preventing the premature deaths of perhaps millions of innocent people (see Ruan & Chong, 1987).

By quoting their letters here, the author has had the good fortune of allowing China's gay people to speak for themselves. There is little doubt that further studies should be conducted to present a more complete picture of homosexuality in China. It is not clear how representative these letter writers are of the gay population. Despite the diversity in terms of age, geographic distribution, and occupations, it is possible that many of the less educated and illiterate may not be represented in this group. We have learned something about how they think and live, but nothing that helps answer such interesting questions as the nature of the relationship between sociocultural background and sexuality.

From a sexological point of view, it is also important to learn more about gay experience in China to improve our knowledge of the cross-cultural characteristics of homosexuality.

FEMALE HOMOSEXUALITY

As noted in the introduction to the previous section on male homosexuality, homosexuality is virtually a forbidden topic in China. Few academic papers on the subject have been published either in Chinese or in Western languages. Recent articles in English by Ruan and Chong (1987) and Ruan and Tsai (1987, 1988) discuss only male homosexuality in mainland China, and articles on lesbianism restrict their discussion to the situation in Hong Kong (Lieh-Mak, O'Hoy, & Luk, 1983; Norrgard, 1990). As of this writing, no academic paper on lesbianism in mainland China has been published in either Chinese or English.

This section begins with a historical survey of lesbianism in Chinese culture and an analysis of the treatment of lesbianism in classical Chinese literature. Next, literary and scholarly materials describing the sexual behaviors of Chinese lesbians are surveyed. Finally, we report the current situation of lesbians in mainland China, based on interviews the senior author conducted in 1985 with young women incarcerated in the Shanghai Women Delinquents Correction Institution, and on several new publications in literary fields in Chinese in mainland China in 1987–1989.

Historical Outline of Lesbianism in China

In ancient times Chinese culture was characterized by a very tolerant attitude toward lesbianism. One important reason was that women's supply of Yin (the substance and/or energy which is essential for the body) was believed to be unlimited in quantity; from this point of view, female masturbation would be harmless. It was also recognized that when a number of women are obliged to live in continuous and close proximity, as did many women living in polygamous households, there are many opportunities for lesbian relationships to develop. Many considered such relationships inevitable, certainly to be tolerated and, according to some, even encouraged. "The Paired Dance of the Female Blue Phoenixes," Posture No. 15 in the noted sex handbook *Book of the Mystery-Penetrating Master* (Tung-hsuan-tzu), gave instructions for a method that not only allowed a man to enjoy two women at once, but simultaneously permitted pleasurable genital contact between the women:

A man and two women: One woman lies on her back with her legs raised. The second woman lies on top of the first, facing her. Their two vaginas face each other. The man sits cross-legged, displaying his jade object (penis), and attacks the vaginas above and below. (Yeh, 1914)

The Chinese use the picturesque term, "mojingzi" (rubbing mirrors, or mirror grinding) to describe lesbian sexual behavior. The image of two flat, mirrorlike surfaces in contact, without any intervening "stemlike" projection (such as the penis) effectively conveys the idea of genital contact between two women. Yao (1941) uses the related term "mojingzhe" (mirror rubbers) to mean "lesbians," offering the following definition: "Two women who are aroused by sexual desires, and having no help, rub their mons pubis for each other."

In modern times, we find examples of formal associations of lesbians. One such organization, the "Mojing Dang" ("Rubbing-mirrors Party") was active in Shanghai in the late nineteenth century. It was said to be a descendant of the "Ten Sisters," which a Buddhist nun had founded several hundred years earlier in Chaozhou, Guangdong (Canton) province. Members of the "Ten Sisters" lived together as couples. The refused to marry, and some even avoided marriage by committing suicide. A few are rumored to have killed their husbands so that they could maintain their lesbian relationships. The nineteenth-century Rubbing-mirrors Party was also led by a Cantonese woman and lasted about twenty years. It had approximately twenty members, including three who were mistresses of wealthy men, one who had never married, and more than a dozen rich widows. They attracted new members through their knowledge of sexual technique.

Chen (1928) describes the "Jinglanhui" (Golden Orchid Association) which was active in the Cantonese counties Shunte, Fanyu, and Sajiao. The membership of this association was exclusively female. Some members lived together as couples for their entire lives. Others married, but continued their lesbian relationships after marriage, avoiding their husbands' homes as much as possible. Some who were forced to stay with their husbands committed suicide. The folklore text *Gazetteer of Chinese Customs* (Zhonghua Chuanguo Fengsu Shi), published in 1935, described the Golden Orchid Association as follows:

> Whenever two members of the association developed deep feelings for each other, certain rites of "marriage" were performed. For such a "marriage" to be permitted, one partner was designated the "husband." The first step consisted of offering to the intended partner a gift of peanut candies, honey, and other sweets. Once this was accepted, a night-long celebration attended by mutual female friends followed. From then on the couple would live as "man and wife." Sexual behaviors like genital contact called "grinding bean curd" or the use of dildos were practiced. The couple could also adopt female

children and these children could inherit the property of their "parents." (Cited by Lieh-Mak, O'Hoy, & Luk, 1983)

The most recent account of female homosexuality in China describes the lesbian subculture in Hong Kong (Norrgard, 1990). These women adopt "male" and "female" roles in a manner reminiscent of the "butch and femme" roles of some American lesbians. Those in the woman's role are expected to passively await for the approaches of those in the man's role. If a woman in the female role takes the initiative, potential partners will avoid her, and all the lesbians in her circle will condemn her. Everyone must know clearly which role each individual will play, and each individual must act within her role. Norrgard has also heard rumors of secret societies of lesbians meeting in Beijing.

Lesbianism in Chinese Literature

The general tolerance of female homosexuality was reflected in ancient Chinese literature, which provides numerous accounts of such relationships. Lesbian relationships were not only portrayed as common and often inevitable; they were known to give rise to beautiful acts of love, self-sacrifice, and devotion, and such acts were praised and celebrated. At the same time, it was believed that excesses should be avoided. Feng Meng-lung (1574–1646), editor of the famous collection of Ming dynasty tales, Stories to Awaken Men (Hsin-Shih Heng-Yen), chose to include the cautionary tale, "King Hailing Dies of Sexual Addiction." In this story, women are punished, perhaps not so much for their lesbian behavior as for rebellion and intrigue.

This story of palace intrigue and revenge portrays the Jin dynasty King Hailing (ruled 1149–1160) as a sexually obsessed man, with many concubines to satisfy his appetites. One of his favorites was Ali Hu, a beautiful woman who had been married three times and was herself unusually eager for sex. The king and Ali Hu enjoyed a wonderful sexual relationship until the day Hailing saw Ali Hu's pretty teenage daughter, Ali Zhongjie, and decided to seduce her. First he tried to arouse her by having her witness a nude sex party, then he entered her bedroom and forced her to have intercourse with him. Hailing became so infatuated with Zhongjie he neglected Hu. Hu, jealous of her daughter and sexually starved, allowed herself to be seduced by a maid-in-waiting. Hu's waitress Shengge, a girl who wore man's clothing according to the requirements of the king's palace, presented Hu with a sex toy, "Mr. Horn" (Chinese dildo). Hu and Shengge enjoyed each other nightly. Then San Niang, a kitchen maid, informed on Shengge, telling the king that

Shengge might really be male and was engaging in adultery with Hu. Because the king had had intercourse with Shengge himself, he knew beyond doubt that she was a woman. Hu killed San Niang, Shengge committed suicide, and eventually Hu was killed by the king.

A more typical, positive portrayal of lesbianism, and the best-known example, is the stage play *Loving the Fragrant Companion* (Lien-hsiang-pan), written by the well-known Ming author Li Yu (1611–1680). Lesbian love is the main theme of the work. At the beginning of the play, young Mrs. Shih visits a temple, where she meets a beautiful and talented young girl called Yun-hua. The two fall passionately in love, and Mrs. Shih promises that she will do her best to make Yun-hua her husband's concubine, so that they can always be together. After many tribulations Mrs. Shih's scheme succeeds, and Mr. Shih is as delighted as his wife. The play is replete with beautiful poetry, and the dialogues—especially those between the two women—are considered brilliant.

While the famous Ching dynasty author Pu Sung-ling (1640–1715) describes a lesbian love relationship of great depth in the story "Fung San Niang" (contained in Volume 5 of Liao-chai chih-i—*Tales of the Unusual from the Leisure Studio*), the most positive story about female homosexuality may be the one told in the famous novel, *Dream of the Red Chamber*. It is the story of two actresses—Ou-kuan, who specializes in male roles, and Di-kuan, who specializes in female roles. These women love each other as passionately in reality as they do onstage. When Di-kuan dies, her "male" partner Ou-kuan is desolated. When the novel's hero Jia Bao-yu learns of the tragedy, he comforts Ou-kuan and encourages her to burn incense in her lover's memory. Jia Bao-yu's gesture shows just how well lesbianism was accepted by the ancient Chinese.

Some painters also depicted lesbian sexual behavior. For example, reproductions can be found in *Erotic Aspects of Chinese Culture* (Girchner, 1957, p. 94).

Sexual Behavior of Chinese Lesbians

Besides describing the social and emotional contexts of female homosexuality, Chinese literature is rich in fictional and nonfictional accounts of explicitly sexual behavior. In his *The Classic of the Human Mirror* (Ren Jing Jing), written in 1641, Zhang Jun-ying reported that he had witnessed two women having orgasms during sexual intercourse. Unfortunately, while he gave detailed descriptions of heterosexual intercourse and male homosexual intercourse, he merely stated that lesbian sexual behavior resembled heterosexual intercourse. Another seventeenthcenturyauthor, using the pen name Siqao Qushi, gave a detailed, evocative description of lesbian seduction and pleasure in his erotic novel *The Flower's Shadow Behind the Curtain* (Ge Lian Hua Ying). In Chapter 22 he wrote:

> Two 16-year-old girls, Dangui and Xiangyu, slept together in one bed. At first, they felt ashamed whenever they touched each other's bodies. After several nights, they began to kiss each other as a man kisses a woman, passionately and shamelessly. One night, they secretly watched their mothers having sex with an old man. Seeing this three-way sexual interaction left them highly excited. As a result, they took off all their clothes and pretended to be a couple making love.
>
> First, Dangui, the elder girl, took the part of the "man." She told Xiangyu, "We may not have a penis as a man does, but we can use our fingers just like a penis." Dangui raised Xiangyu's legs, kissed and sucked her nipples, and touched her vulva. She tried to insert her finger into Xiangyu's vagina, but not even her little finger could get in. She wet her finger with her saliva, and finally succeeded in inserting it into Xiangyu's vagina. At first, the thrusting of Dangui's finger was painful to Xiangyu, but after many thrusts, Xiangyu felt excitement and pleasure. She applauded Dangui, calling her "my darling brother."
>
> At the same time, Xiangyu began caressing Dangui's vulva, and was startled to find it very wet. She asked Dangui, "Why did you urinate?" Dangui replied, "This is women's sexual secretion, and tomorrow when I play with you, you will get as wet as I am." After this, the girls made love every night; each one taking the man's role in turn. Later they made a false penis out of a white silk belt stuffed with cotton. They used it every night for their sexual pleasure. (Siqao, 1987; author's translation)

The exchange of active and passive roles described in Siqao's story is an interesting contrast to the adoption of fixed roles by some lesbians in modern Hong Kong.

The literature describes a variety of means for achieving mutual satisfaction. In addition to such obvious methods as massage, mutual masturbation, cunnilingus, and so forth, a lesbian couple could use artificial aids. An example was the double olisbos, a short ribbed stick made of wood or ivory, with two silk bands attached to the middle. Some medical books warn against excessive use of artificial aids, claiming that they might damage "the lining of the womb." *Important Matters of the Jade Chamber* contains such a warning, and quotes Peng the Methuselah as saying, "The reason that lechery causes you to be short-lived is not always because of the actions of demons and spirits. Women who insert powder into their vaginas or make a male stalk out of ivory and use it always injure their lives and quickly age and die" (translated by Ishihara & Levy, 1968).

The Current Situation of Lesbians in Mainland China

Lesbians in China are even more closeted than gay males. When the author received letters from homosexuals all over China in 1985 and 1986, not one was from a woman. Most of the case reports given here were gleaned from several sensationalistic publications appearing in mainland China from 1987 to 1989. Some of these reports may be distorted, but they do represent the kind of information that is available to the Chinese people, and their preconceptions about lesbians.

By 1990, the situation was unchanged. Lenore Norrgard, a Seattle-based freelance writer who has been active in the lesbian/gay/bisexual and feminist movements since 1975, speaks Chinese, and frequently writes about China, found that she had to focus most of her research on Chinese lesbians on those in Hong Kong. She explains:

> In nearly ten years of visiting, studying, working, and living in China and Hong Kong, I had never managed to meet any women who identified as lesbians. It wasn't because I didn't look: Whenever I got on a conversational basis with someone who seemed relatively open or enlightened, I would ask about homosexuality. (Norrgard, 1990)

Norrgard reports that the usual response was one of "incredible" ignorance and naïveté. While she found the lack of homophobia refreshing, she also noted that in China it is considered "scandalous" even for a married couple to hold hands in public, attributing the lack of awareness of homosexuality to a general lack of sexual knowledge. While studying in Beijing, she did hear of two young women who went to the Marriage Bureau to register their bond, and were promptly arrested. She remarked, "Homosexuality is illegal in China, yet ignorance about it is so vast that the two apparently were not even aware of the taboo" (Norrgard, 1990).

Ignorance, if not repression, is equally widespread in Hong Kong, according to Choi Wan, a 36-year-old lesbian journalist who lives in Hong Kong and belongs to the Association for the Advancement of Feminism. Choi told Norrgard (1990), "In China they're especially naive about lesbianism. Homosexuality among men they can understand more, because it's more often represented in stories. You never read about women having relationships with women."

Some of the women who are willing to discuss their homosexuality have already been imprisoned and have little to lose. The author of this book, as an expert and leading sexologist in China, was the main speaker at the first national workshop on sex education held in Shanghai in August 1985. There he received an invitation from the Shanghai Public Security Bureau to visit the Shanghai Women Delinquents Correction Institution. As the correction officer's counselor, he was asked to interview three women. Two of them, Ms. L. and Ms. Zu, were prostitutes who were described in Chapter 5, and the third, Ms. Za, was a "sex criminal."

Ms. Za was 26 years old, born into an intellectual's family. Her first sexual encounter, with a male classmate, occurred while she was still in high school. She enjoyed sex very much, and had sex with about 30 different men altogether, never taking any money. Because of her sexual "delinquency," she was jailed many times. During one jail term, Ms. Za shared a room with Ms. X, who had been arrested and jailed for lesbian behavior. Ms. Za had never even heard of homosexuality before she met Ms. X. In jail, Ms. X treated Ms. Za like a lover, touching her, petting her, and telling her that even without a man two women can have very good sex. After her initial surprise, Ms. Za greatly enjoyed receiving manual and oral sexual caresses from Ms. X. Later, Ms. Za actively seduced other women. She felt that orgasms resulting from homosexual sex were as strong as those from heterosexual sex, though she preferred male partners. Now, Ms. Za began receiving jail sentences for homosexual "sex crimes," as well as heterosexual promiscuity.

Another case was reported by attorney Dun Li. He represented Ms. Jia, who had been deeply in love with another young woman, Ms. Yi. They were constant companions, fond of calling each other "sister," and shared a bed all night as often as they could manage. Jia had been married 6 months, reluctantly having intercourse with her husband. She only wanted to have sex with Miss Yi. Later, Miss Yi became engaged, but before the wedding, Jia killed her. In court, Jia confessed that she loved Yi so intensely that she wanted to divorce her husband and live with Yi forever. When Yi disagreed, Jia decided that it was better to die herself after killing her lover (Ruan, 1985).

An exception to the usual difficulty in locating lesbians was the experience of Chinese journalists He and Fang (1989), who were actually more successful in contacting lesbians than gay males in their 1989 survey of homosexuality in China. They wrote six stories about lesbians compared to one about gay males. Their stories are summarized here:

> In the autumn of 1988, in a factory in "C" city, Miss Wang, an engineer, used strong acid to burn her colleague and homosexual partner Miss Li, both to prevent and to take revenge for Li's plans to marry a man.

Miss Liu is a very attractive 24-year-old woman who has never had any sexual interest in men. She is a noted fashion designer, who is in love with her sister's friend Miss Zhang, a college student. Miss Zhang reciprocated from the beginning, and the two women (virgins in terms of heterosexual contact) enjoyed a mutually satisfactory sexual relationship. When Liu's mother accidentally discovered her daughter's lesbian relationship, she and her husband forced her to go to the hospital to seek a "cure" for her "disease."

In "B" city, where more than 200 prostitutes had been forced to return from Kuangzhou (Canton), a policeman discovered that two of them were a lesbian couple. Miss Tu was a 22-year-old woman who said her first sexual experience occurred at a sex party where pornographic videotapes were shown; Miss Cheng was a 21-year-old woman who had been a virgin until three men raped her. These two women met by chance in Kuangzhou, where they shared a hotel room. One night, a customer who was an impotent sadist, asked to hire Miss Tu and Miss Cheng together. He ordered them to stimulate each other manually and orally while he watched. This was the first time they had done anything like this, and to their surprise, it gave them much pleasure. After that, they became intimate lovers.

Mr. Wu was a worker who was still single at 30; he had trouble finding a wife because he was so short, but finally he was introduced to Miss Xia. On their wedding night, another woman, Miss Jiang, roughly knocked on the door of the new couple's bedroom. Jiang was Xia's lover, and refused to accept the marriage unless Mr. Wu would agree to take both of them as wives, so the lesbian relationship could be maintained. Jiang forced Mr. Wu to have intercourse with her first, with his new wife Xia second, and then to join them in a menage à trois. Xia was displeased by the good sexual relationship that formed between Wu and Jiang, and reported it to the authorities. Wu was arrested, and Xia and Jiang were forced to separate.

In "Y" county, in the Moon Buddhist Nunnery, there were more than 30 nuns. One day, a very beautiful girl, Miss Wang, insisted on becoming a nun, cutting her long hair herself. Miss Wang took the Buddhist name Huimei, and became the lover of another nun, Huiming. Huiming's former lesbian lover, another nun named Huiyuan, was jealous and broke in on Huiming and Huimei while they were making love. When she broke the door down, their secret came out. Huiming and Huimei had to leave the nunnery and were no longer allowed to be nuns. Huiming said that it was other, older nuns who had originally seduced her.

Miss A was unmarried at 37, and had always been attracted to other women, not men. Finally, she met Miss B, and they became lovers. Even after B's marriage, the two women remained lovers. B's husband was completely ignorant of the situation; he thought Miss

A visited the house so frequently because she wanted to have an affair with him! (He & Fang, 1989)

He and Fang encountered the usual reluctance to be interviewed among people who had every reason to fear discovery. They, too, had to rely on interviews with women who were jailed for "sex crimes," or crimes of violence inspired by sexual jealousy. Because so many investigations of female homosexuality are based on interviews with prisoners, it has been all too easy for Chinese people to develop a stereotype of lesbians as immoral, frustrated people. Thus Shui (1989), in an article in which it is impossible to separate fact from fiction, describes a secret "Lesbians' Company" of women who engage in murder and other crimes because they have been hurt and rejected by men. Unfortunately, this story, one of the few publications in which homosexuality in mainland China has been discussed, is probably representative of common attitudes toward lesbianism.

Perhaps a more representative story is one that was told to Wan Ruixiong. The interviewee had only been married a short time when, in 1957, her husband was accused of "Rightism," and sent to a forced-labor camp. Soon after the arrest, their son was born, and not long after that, the father died of starvation. The woman, who never did remarry, lived in extreme poverty. One day another woman visited her, bringing food. Eventually they became lovers, and have enjoyed a pleasurable sexual relationship for many years.

It is clear that many Chinese lesbians do live painful lives, marred by fear and jealousy. But it is impossible to develop a complete and balanced picture of their lives under current conditions.

No national or local statistics about homosexuals in China are available, and the kind of formal, broad survey that could develop such statistics cannot be made under prevailing repressive policies. Even anecdotal evidence must be distorted when the majority of those who supply it do so only because they are coerced by legal authorities. Given the general lack of sex information in China, and the repressive attitudes of the leadership, it will be a long time before Chinese homosexuals can hope to live normal, fulfilling lives.

Transvestism and Transsexualism

TRANSVESTISM

The term "transvestism" has been given different definitions by different authors. For example, Hyde (1982) says, "Transvestism refers to dressing as a member of the opposite gender," while Strong and DeVault (1988) narrow the definition by stating, "Transvestites are men who wear women's clothes or garments in order to become sexually aroused." Our discussion will apply the broadest definition of transvestism—that is, any instance of men or women dressing in the clothing of the opposite sex—including as a subcategory those "true transvestites" who are sexually aroused by the practice.

There is almost no material in English about transvestism in China. For example, van Gulik's *Sexual Life in Ancient China* contains no mention of transvestism or transvestites in either the index or the text. In modern Chinese literature, not a single research article on transvestism in China is to be found. Except for a few examples cited from English books about transvestism, most of the material surveyed here was translated by the author from Chinese texts. These materials are used as the basis for a classification of types of transvestism according to the motivation for the practice.

Historical Accounts of Transvestism in Ancient China

The first recorded case of transvestism was that of Meixi, the concubine of King Xia Jie (about 1600 B.C.). She was a strikingly beautiful woman who enjoyed dressing in men's clothing and wearing a sword (Samshasha, 1984).

The writings of Hsun Kung (ca. 313–238 B.C.) showed that male transvestism—and disapproval of the practice—existed more than 2,000 years ago: "There was a bad custom of many men dressing like women in very beautiful fashions. Their voice, action, and attitude imitated women also. Even women were eager to marry them" (cited in Jiang, 1988).

Another female transvestite was the famous and powerful empress Wu Tse-tian (A.D. 624–705). In her childhood, she dressed as a boy. During her reign (A.D. 690–705), she wore the male imperial costume, and her male sexual partners dressed like female concubines (Samshasha, 1984).

Some records suggest that while some transvestism may have been protected by imperial privilege, the situation for commoners may have been different. *History of the Southern Dynasties from A.D. 420–589* (Nan Shih) recorded the case of Zheng Lou, a woman who left her native town of Dongyang dressed as a man and became an officer in Yangzhou. When it was discovered that the officer was a woman, the emperor Mingti (reigned A.D. 562–585) ordered her to return to Dongyang dressed as a woman (Weixing, 1984).

Classification with Examples of Transvestism in China

There have been numerous motivations for cross dressing in China, especially in ancient China.

For Male Prostitution

The noted Southern Sung writer Chou Mi (1232–1308) recorded that in the Wu Area, where male prostitutes were very common, they frequented the Xinmenwai district made up very much like women and dressed in beautiful feminine fashion. They were said to sew as well as any woman and used women's names. (Guixin zashi [*The Guixin Miscellanies*], cited in Samshasha, 1989). According to the famous Ching dynasty scholar Chao I (1727–1814), these men, who even had a professional guild, were continuing a practice that had been common in the preceding Northern Sung dynasty (960–1127). In fact, during the Cheng-ho era (1111–1117) a law was promulgated which prescribed a penalty of 100 blows with a bamboo rod, a heavy punishment for male prostitution (van Gulik, 1961).

As was discussed in Chapter 7, during the Chien Lung and Chia Ching periods of the Ching dynasty (A.D. 1736–1820), the popular phrase "shiahng gung" was used at various times in reference to male actors who played female characters, any male actors who took the "female" role in homosexual relations, or male homosexual prostitutes. They dressed as women, wore perfume and cosmetics, and even moved like women; the slang phrase "shiahng gu" had the flavor of the American expressions "drag queen" and "hustler." In Beijing, where the practice flourished, houses of male prostitution were called "shiahng-gung tang-sze."

For Professional Purposes

Although the same terminology was sometimes applied to both homosexuals and to actors who played female roles, such usage may not have been meant literally. The famous Peking Opera, an intricate form of theater combining song, dance, pantomime, and acrobatics, originally resembled the theater of Shakespeare's time in that all roles, both male and female, were played by men. When women entered the theater, they sometimes took male roles, and the practice of men playing female roles continued. Even after the founding of the People's Republic of China, some of the most famous players in the Peking theater were men who acted in female roles. One of them, Mei Lanfang (1894–1961), was not only the most prominent star, but the first to introduce Peking Opera to foreign audiences, visiting Japan, the Soviet Union, and the United States. In America, he received an enthusiastic reception and critical acclaim, and his makeup, facial expression, and falsetto singing voice were all highly praised for their unearthly beauty (Wu, Huang, & Mei, 1981).

Less famous than the Peking Opera, which tours all China, is the younger, more regional Shaoxing Opera. This theater has a tradition opposite to that of the Peking Opera: all roles, both male and female, are played by women.

For Economic Purposes

There are a number of accounts of young boys being sold as girls because that would bring the seller a higher profit. Often they were sold as children, and sometimes the deception was not discovered until they were old enough to be taken as concubines. These incidents occurred in several different eras.

A Ching dynasty (1644–1911) writer described such a story in detail:

> A person brought a ten-year-old girl to sell in Beijing. A scholar called Shutang Xu paid 30,000 coins and bought her to be his waitress. Xu called her Lihua (Pear Flower). Later Lihua became a very beautiful young lady. Her makeup was so pretty, no other woman

could compare with her. When Xu's daughter married, Lihua was appointed as one of the two concubines to accompany Xu's daughter in marriage. [This was a custom in the feudal marriage system of imperial China.] The bridegroom of these three women loved Lihua very much and tried many times to have sex with her. But Lihua avoided it as well as she possibly could. When their family went on a journey by ship, one night an assistant of the bridegroom's father accidentally saw a beautiful woman standing up on the side of the third ship to urinate with a big penis. It was Lihua, the eighteen-year-old beauty! Next day, the bridegroom was told of this surprising discovery. The bridegroom closed the door and examined Lihua's sexual organs by force. Eventually, Lihua told the truth, that her parents had been very poor and sold her to survive. "At that time, a girl's price was ten times that of a boy. Therefore, my parents dressed me as a girl to sell to you." (Weixing 1964)

For Access to Social Prerogatives

Chinese literature and folklore are replete with stories of young women who disguised themselves as men so they could gain access to social roles that were otherwise closed to them. In one story so famous that it has been quoted in many Western texts, the legendary heroine Hua Mulan showed her filial devotion by dressing as a man so she could replace her elderly father on the field of battle.

Such stories reflect a social situation in which women could not become soldiers or scholars, or even travel in safety without a male escort. The theme of a woman traveling in male disguise, which is found in the folklore of many such cultures, may reflect real (if uncommon) occurrences.

In one very popular love story, Zhu Yintai, a beautiful girl who lived in Henan during the Spring–Autumn Period (770–221 B.C.), and was sixteen at the time the events of the story unfolded, dressed as a young man to go to a residential school in Hangzhou for better education. There she fell in love with her classmate Liang Shan-pei, who slept with her for a long time without ever recognizing that she was in fact a woman (Wenhua, 1984).

Another such tale is found in a famous short story in *Stories to Awaken Men*. According to this tale, there was a very kind, rich, and childless old man who, at different times and in different circumstances, had adopted two young men. After the old man passed away, the adopted brothers did business together very successfully. Many families tried to marry their daughters to these brothers. But the younger brother always rejected every offer, and even opposed marriage for his older brother. At last the younger brother wrote two poems to tell the older brother that "he" was in fact a young lady, who had disguised herself as a young man in order to travel in safety and then had been adopted as the old man's "son." The two who had loved each other as brothers married and became a very happy couple (Feng, 1981).

For Sexual Deception

Ancient Chinese literature contains many tales of men who dressed as females so that they could gain access to women for purposes of rape or seduction. There are also records of actual incidents of this nature.

In A.D. 1465 a resident of Taidung named Gu Zai was sentenced to death for raping several women after he had entered their bedrooms dressed as a woman. He was even teaching his methods to a young man named San Zung.

Perhaps the most spectacular case, recorded in several histories, is that of Sang Chong. He was the adopted son of Mao Sang of Yuci county of Sanxi province. From childhood, he dressed as a girl, even binding his feet. As an adult, he became a "seamstress," which gave him access to many families and the opportunity to rape 182 women in 45 counties over the course of 10 years. He was finally discovered on July 13, 1476, when a young man attempted to rape him and discovered his true sex.

To the extent that such practices really occurred, they may have continued into the twentieth century. The Bailian jiao (White Lotus Society), a secret sect which was active during the Ming and Ching dynasties (1368–1911), was rumored to have many members who dressed as women so they could have sexual adventures (Weixing, 1964).

In *Tales of the Unusual from the Leisure Studio* (Liao-chai chih-i), Pu Sung-ling told such a story:

> Wanbao Ma and his wife Tian were both very lustful, and they had a very good relationship. She helped him use a trick to sleep with a beautiful lady who was living in their neighborhood as a guest and tailor. He found that this lady was a man in woman's clothing, and he cut off "her" penis, taking her as his partner for anal sex for the rest of their lives. (Weixing, 1964)

A variation on the theme was the use of female disguise to conceal adulterous relationships. Yuan Mei (1715–1797) was unquestionably the most popular writer of the Ching dynasty, one of very few poets to have flourished under Manchu rule (Giles, 1967). In his *New Tales*, originally titled *What the Master Would Not Talk Of* (Zibuyu), Yuan told this story:

> In Guiyang county, a beautiful man named Hong dressed in woman's clothes and worked as a tailor, teaching his trade to ladies in Hubei and Guizhou provinces. A young scholar from Changsa,

Li, hired "her" to do some embroidery, then tried to seduce "her."
When Hong told him the truth, Li said with a smile, "Are you really
a man? That is wonderful, even much better than a woman for me.
I always thought that the King of Northern Wei (386–557) was very
foolish that when he saw his mother accompanied by two beautiful
nuns, and when he had sex with them and discovered that they were
male, had them arrested and punished. The king should have let
them become his homosexual partners. If he had done so, he would
have brought himself a great deal of sexual happiness without hurt-
ing his mother in any way." Hong accepted Li's viewpoint, and became Li's lover.

Several years later, Hong went to Jingxia. There a man named
Tu wanted to have sex with Hong, who he supposed was a beautiful
woman. When Tu discovered Hong's male organ, Tu rejected him
and Hong was arrested. Hong revealed that as an orphan he had
been adopted by a widow and had a sexual relationship with her.
She had him dress as a girl so they could avoid discovery. After the
widow died, when Hong was seventeen, he kept his disguise, going
out to work as a tailor. For the next ten years, until he was arrested,
he had sex with many women. (Weixing, 1964; author's translation)

For Superstitious Reasons

Apparently some families disguised their male children as females
to protect them from harm. This was the history of the Ching Dynasty
poet Miengu. None of his older brothers had survived, and an astrologer
advised his parents to protect their next son by dressing him as a girl.
Miengu enjoyed the female role, married a rather masculine woman, and
dressed his own sons like girls.

True Transvestism

A "true" transvestite is one who derives sexual gratification from
cross dressing. If there have been any true transvestites in China, they
have been so secretive that not one case has been recorded in ancient or
contemporary Chinese literature. It is remarkable that there are materials
about homosexuality, transsexualism, exhibitionism, fetishism, bestiality,
necrophilia, sadism and masochism, pedophilia, incest, and other variations in sexual behavior in China, yet nothing about transvestism. Possibly some transvestites in the above categories actually enjoyed cross
dressing also, but their true motives were disguised. Also, transvestites
who do not feel "ill" or "abnormal," and therefore do not seek medical
or psychiatric attention, will remain undiscovered. It is true that the uni-
sexual costume which now prevails in mainland China decreases the

motivation for cross dressing. Yet it is difficult to imagine that a practice which occurs in so many other cultures does not also occur in China. If the current sexual repression in China is lifted, authentic reports of transvestism may appear in the near future.

TRANSSEXUALISM

Recognition of transsexualism in human society is a relatively recent phenomenon. The term was not even coined until 1949, and did not come into widespread use until the 1960s.

Transsexuals represent a small proportion of any population. According to a recent estimate (Sierles, 1982), male transsexuals number 1 in every 40,000–100,000, and female transsexuals are even fewer, numbering about 1 in every 100,000–400,000. While there have been numerous studies about transsexualism in the West, none has been conducted in China. China's population of 1.1 billion—one quarter of the world's population—and distinctive historical and cultural traditions make the question of whether transsexualism exists there an interesting one. Also, if transsexualism does exist in China, is it similar to that in the West?

An Analysis of Transsexuals in China

Data and Methods

In 1982, the author had a column, "Psychological Counseling," in China's widely read popular medical magazine, *To Your Good Health*. It was the first of its kind in mainland China and was very well received. Not surprisingly, a wide variety of questions about the personal problems of readers and their acquaintances were received from all over the country. By the end of 1985, seven letters had been sent by self-described transsexuals, some of whom described themselves and their problems in great detail. Two of these men corresponded with the author several times, even enclosing photographs which revealed some of their unique physical characteristics. In fact, the author performed a medical examination of one of them, and eventually helped him find a surgeon to conduct sex-change surgery.

A content analysis of these 16 letters received from seven Chinese transsexuals provides an initial description of transsexualism in contemporary mainland China (Ruan & Bullough, 1988; Ruan, Bullough, & Tsai, 1989).

Results

General Characteristics.   All seven of these Chinese transsexuals are male. Each expressed a strong desire to be a woman. Their ages at the time their letters were written were 20, 19, 23, and 20, respectively (two did not specify their ages but said that they were less than 30 years old).

Their residences, educational levels, and occupations suggest that transsexuals are distributed throughout China, both geographically and socially. One did not mention where he lived; the others lived in Beijing, Qinhai, Jiangxi, Hubei, and Sichuan. Two did not mention their occupations; the others included one business manager, one college student, two workers, and one farmer. One was a college graduate, two were vocational high school graduates, one was a general high school graduate, and while the rest did not mention their educational status, their letters suggested that they had at least some high school education.

Five of the seven used their real names and addresses from the beginning, while two used pseudonyms and, at first, referred to themselves in the third person. Their caution was understandable, given the social pressures against transsexualism. Because of their need for anonymity, all seven will be referred to by case number.

Two of the seven dressed and lived as women all the time, and only one, 7, was married. He wrote, "I have been married for several years. My wife is with me but I cannot free myself of the strong psychological desire to be a woman. I would rather masturbate than have a sexual relationship with my wife."

Some Typical Chinese Transsexual Cases

Some of the letters provided detailed descriptions of the experiences, psychological development, and emotional lives of their authors. Their stories seem to typify the lives of Chinese transsexuals.

Case 1 is 20 years old. Medical examination found that both his external sex organs and his sex chromosomes were those of a normal male. His parents treated him as a girl so that he would not fight or soil his clothes. He was dressed like a girl until he was about thirteen or fourteen years old, when he entered junior high school. His parents forced him to dress like a boy after that, but he did not want to. He became very quiet and isolated from his peers. He could not forget about his colorful girl's clothing. His parents sent him to join the army hoping that he would become more masculine. He recalled:

In the military, everybody ate, slept, and bathed in the same open facilities. It was frightening to me. I was so afraid that I dared not to go to the bathroom and could not sleep well at night.

His desire to change his identity and return to women's clothing was so strong that he threatened to commit suicide. He was finally permitted to leave the military and returned to his preferred (women's) clothing, identity, and way of life. He took stilbestrol for more than a year. As a result, his breasts enlarged and his body structure and appearance, voice and mannerisms became more feminine. His appearance was that of a beautiful, rather docile woman. His employer fell in love with him and wanted to marry him, insisting even after he revealed his true identity. He considered himself no different from a normal woman and was strongly attracted to men. He felt that his was an ordinary feminine libido, and said that he disliked homosexuality. He had a strong, persistent desire to be a woman and marry a man, and said that he would rather die than live as a man.

In January 1983, with the author's assistance, he underwent transsexual surgery in the Plastic Surgery Department of the Third Hospital of Beijing Medical University. His penis and testes were removed and a vagina was made. The surgery was a complete success. He is one of the few known successful transsexuals in modern mainland China.

Case 1's story seems to suggest that gender reversal in childhood can lead to transsexualism. However, his older brother was also raised as a girl at first, and had little trouble reversing his gender identity later. Evidently, mistaken gender socialization alone is not sufficient to cause transsexualism.

Case 2 wrote:

> I am a strange young man. I constantly want to be a woman. This is because everything about me, such as my hobbies, personality, looks, and especially my psychological activity (dreams and fantasies), typifies a young woman. Like most young women, I dream and fantasize about being married to a suitable husband, not to an able and kind wife. In any event, inside I'm 100 percent woman. I cannot change this mentality. I feel like the same sex/gender as women, and like men are the opposite sex from me. But my sex organ is male. This contradiction between my body and my mind tortures me constantly.
>
> I once had a girl friend but, because I'm a woman inside, I could not bring myself to love her or any woman. I am deeply in love with a man right now. Because of my personal character, looks, orientation, and my tender and passionate personality, he loves me just as much. But he thinks I'm like Zhu Yintai [the aforementioned woman who dressed as a man in a story famous in traditional Chinese fiction and

drama]. The pain inside me is beyond description. I don't dare tell him the truth about myself, or I might lose him. I contemplated suicide often, then thought about not being even 20 years old, and stopped. I wish I could rid myself of this horrifying problem. I do not want much. If I could just cut off my sex organ and live, work, and study as a woman, even without marriage, I would be extremely satisfied. I could bear physical pain, but the mental and psychological anguish are truly unbearable. I am in pain, yet I have no one to turn to. Nobody knows how much I suffer. I can only sigh to this emptiness. I often stand looking out the window and cry. I even cry in my dreams. My pain and suffering are worse than those who experience problems or broken hearts in their love life. Everyone can get what they want: a man as a man and a woman as a woman. I can get neither. Because of my strong female psychological orientation I am very secretive about going to the bathroom or taking a shower. I am living in deep anguish and pain daily.

The author suggested that Case 2 seek to have transsexual surgery performed at one of the three large hospitals in the largest city of his home province. These hospitals were well equipped to perform this type of surgery, but he was repeatedly refused. This is typical of the problems faced by transsexuals in China today.

Case 5 wrote:

I am writing to you with pain and sad tears. I hope you can save me. You must find a way to save me. Please, Mr. Kindness, I beg you.

I am 23 years old. My sex organ tells me that I am a man. But my other physical attributes, my mind, thoughts, hobbies, make-up, the way I talk all resemble a genuine young woman. Nobody knows my pain. I dare not go to public bathrooms; instead, I go to the hills or bushes to do these things. I'm too embarrassed to venture out to the public bath house either. Instead I hide in my room and just wipe my body with hot water. Dear Sir, I am afraid to do anything else. If you tried to force a girl to go to the men's room or bath house, she would do exactly what I do.

I have a boy friend. He is handsome, tall, educated, a graduate student pursuing a master's degree. I love him. He loves me even more. We're inseparable. We have never made love. I am what I am, and I'm afraid he'll find out. I am not lying to him; I do it because I love him. I am afraid of losing him. Ever since I can remember I have loved to wear colorful clothing and skirts. I remember wearing my mother's beautiful clothes behind her back. I loved to play with girls and asked them to tie my hair in a pony tail, and wore girls' clothing whenever I could. I didn't want to play with boys. I jumped rope and played girls' games with girls. I went to girls' bathrooms and bath houses.

When I was in elementary school my mother decided that I was too old to go to the girls' bath house. My father took me to the men's bath house once. I remember it was a Saturday. The bath house was very crowded. I was astounded to see so many naked adult men. I was terrified. I've never gone back to a men's public bath house.

In elementary school we did not make gender distinctions so I was able to live and play like a girl. I learned how to knit, sew, and crochet. I was about 8 or 9 years old then.

In junior high school things started to change. We began to make gender distinctions, so I became a loner. Since I loved to study I had very good grades. When I was a freshman in high school, my life took a sharp turn. My neighbor's son transferred from a rural school to my school (in the city). I was called to home the day after his arrival to meet him. His name was S.H. He was tall, strong, and though not full-grown, he was very nice looking. I was introduced to him by his mother as Miss G. She wanted me to look after him since he would be a new student in my school. He was very courteous. He stood up with his shy red face and poured me a cup of tea. I did not know whether I was excited or tense—I couldn't tell. I looked at him passionately.

From that day on we became inseparable. We both got good marks and were promoted to sophomore together. He was four years older than I. Growing up in a rural area had made him very mature and capable. He took good care of me and I helped him in school work and in financial matters. We practiced English conversation and shared difficult school work. I saved all my allowance to buy him books and clothing (his family was very poor). Whenever my family had good food I always saved a big portion for him. He protected me outside the home. Whenever someone was nasty to me he would teach them a lesson so they never tried it again. Gradually we fell deeply in love. When we graduated from high school he passed the college entrance examination to a very famous university, but I failed the test. I couldn't bear this and became quite ill. He stayed by my bedside, caring for me and nurturing me day after day.

The night before he left for college we couldn't bear the idea of separation. We held and embraced each other passionately for a long time. I loved him deeply. He liked me and loved me sincerely. I revealed my deep love to him. He thought I was a hermaphrodite. He said to me, "Q, go to a doctor for treatment. I will love you forever. I can't live without you for even a day." I cried and fell in his arms. Our feeling toward each other increased as time went by. When he graduated from college he continued his study. He is now studying for a master's degree. I went to work in a factory after I graduated from a vocational school. I am now 23 years old and he is 27. It is time to begin a family. I am in deep suffering. I want very strongly to become a woman through surgery. The provincial hospital and my family both object to it. Oh heaven! If I can't have the surgery, I will feel like a person with cancer and die tragically. Dear Mr. Kindness, my life is just beginning. I have a lot I want to do. Please save me. I beg you to find a way for me to have the surgery. I am waiting eagerly for your response.

THE CURRENT SITUATION OF TRANSSEXUALS IN CHINA

Two other cases of transsexualism became known to the author through his efforts to help Case 1. Before undergoing transsexual surgery, Case 1 was examined and treated by a psychiatrist, Dr. H. Y. Yang. Dr. Yang told the author that he had seen two transsexual patients who, after being repeatedly denied transsexual surgery, used knives to remove the penis by themselves.

Of the few published reports of transsexualism in China, most are sensationalistic and condemnatory in tone. Often these stories do not come out until the transsexual, like Dr. Yang's patients, becomes so desperate that he attempts to perform the surgery himself. One such person divorced his wife after introducing her to a suitable partner, applied for surgery several times, and finally made independent arrangements to have his penis and testicles removed (the original report in H. X. Yang, 1988, does not make clear whether the man actually operated on himself). Another went to a public restroom in Hong Kong to operate on himself, and was found with a suicide note in his pocket.

Such desperate acts, and the pleas for help quoted here, are vivid testimony of the existence of transsexuals in mainland China today. Their psychological characteristics and strong desire to have transsexual surgery are exactly the same as those of Western transsexuals. This is evidence that transsexualism itself is not a culture-bound phenomenon.

The greatest difficulty facing transsexuals in modern China is that of gaining the acceptance of their families and society. It is nearly impossible to obtain permission to perform transsexual surgery. The problem is not a lack of appropriate surgical techniques and facilities. In fact, both general plastic surgery and such precise surgical techniques as reimplantation of severed fingers are very advanced in China. If permission were given, transsexual surgery could be performed with little difficulty in most large hospitals.

The problem is really perceptual and ideological. The absence of scientific research on the subject means that there is nothing to counteract the statements of the popular press, which describes transsexualism as not merely outlandish, but as evidence of the inroads of "decadent Western culture." This ideological tone effectively inhibits surgeons' ability to perform transsexual surgery. Anyone who performs this surgery risks being labeled as someone who accepts Western "decadence," a social stigma that is difficult to bear. This situation is an obvious source of conflict for medical professionals, since refusing to perform transsexual surgery in order to relieve the physical and psychological suffering of their patients violates their humanitarian and moral responsibilities.

The courageous confessions of the seven transsexuals who corresponded with the author point to a reality that conflicts with the image demanded by official ideology. One of the most interesting characteristics they share is that not one appears to have had any direct contact with Western culture, let alone the opportunity to be significantly influenced by it. All were born in China after 1949. Some come from rural areas and from the remote region of Northwest China. We must hope that the stories told here will provide some basis for future objective, scientific research on this subject, and that whatever insight has been provided will contribute to better and more complete understanding of this human phenomenon.

Changing Attitudes toward Sex in China Today

STRESS FACTORS: TRADITIONAL CONSERVATISM, OFFICIAL REPRESSION, AND PRIVATE PERMISSIVENESS

For much of China's history, the government was generally lax in enforcing laws pertaining to sexual behavior. Not until the twelfth century, in the Sung dynasty, did the government begin to develop a consistent policy of exercising control over the sexual life of the people, and official constraints on sexual expression developed into a pervasive cultural conservatism. By the beginning of the Ming dynasty, repressive institutions and policies were firmly in place and continued to be in force throughout the Ming and Ching dynasties. Thus, for example, writing about sex, and public discussion of the subject, were forbidden. Strict censorship and other controls persisted after the establishment of the Republic of China in 1912.

Despite the Chinese Communist Party's declared support of women's liberation, little changed after the establishment of Communist rule in 1949. In fact, we may now be witnessing the most repressive period in all Chinese history. The prevailing atmosphere is maintained not only by informal social sanctions, but as a matter of government policy.

The only sexual behavior which is acknowledged to be legally and morally permissible is heterosexual intercourse within a monogamous marriage. Every imaginable variation is explicitly proscribed. Thus prostitution, polygamy, premarital and extramarital intercourse (including cohabitation arrangements), homosexuality, and variant sexual behaviors are all illegal. Because sexual expression is viewed with contempt as the least important activity of life, not only are pornography and nudity banned, but any social activity with sexual implications—such as dancing—may be subject to restrictions. Even the marriage relationship is given little consideration. Thus China's official prudishness and restrictiveness is unrelieved by any appreciation of individual happiness or romantic love.

The pervasive misery produced by these policies is strikingly evident to Western observers. Chou (1971) explicitly compares conditions in China to those during more restrictive periods in the West when he comments, "It is obvious that the life of the ordinary people in China has been governed by a set of rules far more puritanical than any observed by the original Puritans themselves. This is what the Chinese Communists term 'political correctness' regarding one's private life, including sex and love."

John Money (1977), describing a 1974 visit to Peking, showed how the most insignificant encounter is distorted by official prudery: "I came across a slogan: 'Making love is a mental disease that wastes time and energy,' but I could not satisfy myself as to the extent or strength of its impact. It was clearly obvious to me, however, that there was little evidence of romantic love in parks and public places. On a landing of the back stairway of a department store, I happened upon a young couple descending, holding hands. They were as flustered as if I had seen them partly naked."

The conspicuous absence of any expressions of affection that had been noted by Money led Pelton (1982) to remark, "While love and marriage are alive and well in China, sexual activity may be minimal."

Even these perceptive remarks by foreign observers can only hint at the impact of the government's restrictive policies. Indeed, one problem is that an effect of these policies is the creation of difficulties in getting a clear picture of the sexual life of the people. It is evident that government policies oppose the sentiments of significant segments of the population, perhaps a majority in some instances. But, since legal and social sanctions prevent people from expressing their differences openly, much of the evidence is inferential. A detailed description of how some policies are implemented, continuously compared and contrasted with what is known about popular beliefs and practices, may give a clearer impression of their invasive, oppressive character.

The Proscription of Cohabitation and Premarital Sex

The harshness with which these policies have recently been enforced is just one consequence of the tensions resulting from change in response to Western influences. While it may be noted that increasing sexual openness is still a source of tension and unrest in many Western societies, the situation is far more extreme in China, where a more rigid social structure makes change especially stressful. Thus Liu Dalin, a sociologist in Shanghai, has commented, "The Chinese are like people who have been in the dark a long time. Suddenly, when the windows are opened, they feel dizzy" (Burton, 1988). To extend Mr. Liu's analogy, we might add that during repressive eras in the West, considerable light poured in through cracks in the window-frame, whereas in China, the blackout was almost complete.

Then, beginning in the late 1970s, the increased tolerance of nonmarital cohabitation in the West began to influence China's younger generation. College students and young intellectuals in particular were attracted to this life-style. Some of the younger or more open-minded sociologists also asserted the necessity of overcoming the disadvantages of traditional marriage. Actually practicing cohabitation was an act of courage. Unlike Americans dealing with such impediments as reluctant landlords or restrictive zoning ordinances, these young Chinese risked arrest.

In October 1987, for example, 18 couples who were living together in the campus dormitories of Shenzhen University were arrested by campus police. (Shenzhen is a special economic open city near Hong Kong.) Immediately afterward, the University administration announced that all female students living in the women's dormitories must be back in their bedrooms before midnight; otherwise they would not be allowed into the dormitory, and would be expected to give a clear explanation of their absence the following day (*Centre Daily News*, October 26, 1987).

In 1988, in Shanghai, 24-year-old poet Zhang Shaopo was sentenced to 5 years' imprisonment because he organized a sexual-freedom commune with another young man and several young women. All these young persons were living together in one apartment, and none was married. Zhang had graduated from college in Shanghai in 1984, and until 1987 he worked as an editor for a small literary magazine in Jiangsu province. In 1987, he returned to Shanghai, where he worked as a professional poet, and established a commune. In May of 1987, he was arrested. His friends feared that he would be sentenced to death. He was given a lighter sentence only because the women involved refused to accuse him of rape (*Centre Daily News*, March 10, 1988).

These policies are at odds with recent changes of attitude among the Chinese people. In a survey of 23,000 people in 15 provinces conducted by the Shanghai Sex Sociology Research Center in 1989–1990, 86% of the respondents said they approved of premarital sex (Burton, 1990). The study's director, Mr. Liu Dalin, estimates that 30% of China's youth do engage in premarital sex. The tension between realism and moralism is reflected in Mr. Liu's worrying that "If we teach them how to prevent pregnancies, maybe premarital sex will become even more common" (Burton, 1988). There seems little reason to expect that more realistic policies will develop.

What seems to be happening is that premarital intercourse and cohabitation, irregular marriages, and unwanted pregnancies all are increasing. Abortion statistics can give only a partial indication of premarital sexual activity, because some unmarried women claim to be married when they seek abortions, others marry when they learn they are pregnant, and others do not become pregnant. Thus it is highly significant that in a rural (and presumably more conservative) region of Zhejiang province, 66% of unmarried women reportedly have had at least one abortion (*Centre Daily News*, July 25, 1988). It is also significant that the proportion of admittedly unmarried women seeking abortion is increasing. For example, the *Da Gong Daily News* reported on March 22, 1989 that in Shanghai, China's most populous city, the number of abortion patients who said they were unmarried rose from 16% in 1986 to 40% in 1987. The *Centre Daily News* (September 10, 1987) reported that in the central hospital of a large city in Shandong province, at least 38% of the abortions performed in 1985 and 47% of the abortions performed from January to May of 1986 were done for unmarried women. (Since some women who are not married claim that they are, hospital physicians estimate that the true figure may be 50–60%.)

Another survey in the same city in Shandong suggested that 80% of the young women there engage in premarital sex (*Centre Daily News*, September 10, 1987), while a study in a major city in Kuangdong province found that of 123 young women undergoing premarital examinations, 75 (61%) had already experienced intercourse (*Centre Daily News*, July 25, 1988).

The definitions used in compiling official statistics make it difficult to estimate the popularity of unmarried cohabitation in the sense it is understood in the West. The Chinese phrase "weihun tongju," which may be translated as "unmarried cohabitation," includes relationships between couples who are living together without benefit of *both* a government marriage certificate *and* a wedding. The phrase for couples who marry before the legal age (22 for men and 20 for women), "zaohun," again may refer to people who engaged in traditional wedding festivities without benefit of a marriage certificate. There is no difficulty in gathering statistics about these relationships, because generally those responsible for collecting them are local officials and civil servants who, far from being opposed to such marriages, support them for their own families. Still, the official figure of 2.69 million couples in unmarried cohabitation (*Centre Daily News*, April 22, 1989) seems low, considering that some areas report that as many as 50% of couples living together live in unmarried cohabitation. As for couples marrying under the legal age, China's State Family Planning Commission reports that 6.1 million such marriages took place in 1987 alone, and that 2.5 million babies—10% of all births—were born to underage couples in that year; the same news article reports an estimate by the Marriage Administration Division of the National Department of Civil Administration that 30% of China's "married" couples are living together without having received an official marriage certificate, and that the number is growing (*International Daily News*, July 25, 1990). In short, every year there are millions of marriages that are not strictly legal.

Meanwhile, one of the worst aspects of the current law is the potential for repression through selective enforcement. Obviously the government must at least hesitate to jail one-third of its youth. But it can make examples out of people, as in the cases cited earlier, and young people cannot fail to notice that penalizing sexual activities can be a pretext for punishing those who are "troublemakers" in other respects. The fear and circumspection resulting from this situation contribute to maintaining an atmosphere of guilt and ignorance.

Restrictions on Nudity and Depictions of Nudity

The traditional feudal ban on nudity, as maintained by the Chinese Communist Party, is more thoroughgoing than anything currently found in the West. Even if we avoid comparison with the nude beaches of the Riviera, or Danish pornography, and instead compare China with the more conservative United States, the contrast is stark. In the United States, even before the sexual revolution, the naturist movement advocated nude sunbathing as socially and physically healthy, and nudity in the classical arts was fairly well accepted. The Supreme Court doctrine that nudity and sexual activity might be portrayed in a context of "redeeming" social or literary value would be branded self-contradictory by the Chinese government. Similarly, the doctrine of regulation according to prevailing local standards would be rejected because it allows for open—if not always civil—public discussion. In fact, just as conflicting attitudes are held by different segments of the American populace, differences exist among the Chinese; however, the Chinese government consistently endorses and enforces only the most restrictive views.

It is clear that the beauty of the human body holds a great deal of attraction for a significant proportion of the Chinese people. Any magazine or calendar which includes pictures of partially nude women always becomes a kind of best-seller (pictures of completely nude women are almost impossible to publish). Authors, editors, publishers, and readers alike desire such illustrations. Yet the highest political leaders can be relied on always to reprimand publishers and authors for their "vulgar interests."

Even the use of nude models in art colleges has been forbidden. In this instance, even a somewhat progressive attitude by a revered leader may not have overcome traditional resistance. At one time, Mao Tzedong had supported the use of nude models for art instruction. Even so, the artists who used nude models and the nude models themselves faced many difficulties, including outright persecution, as a recent example illustrates.

On February 4 and March 15, 1988, the *Centre Daily News* reported on the story of Chen Suhua who, as a student of nineteen, had posed nude for classes at the Nanjing Art College. In 1986, she became ill and returned from the provincial capital to her native village. The peasants there believed that a nude model is essentially a prostitute and a disgrace to her village. They surrounded Miss Chen's house, insulting her and shouting accusations of prostitution. Eventually, she committed suicide. China's most famous living painter, Professor Wu Zuoren, the president of the Chinese Association of Painters, made a point of telling journalists at an exhibition in Hong Kong how deeply he regretted the fact that such an incident could occur in the 1980s (*Centre Daily News*, February 4, and March 15, 1988).

While such incidents reflect differences among various sectors of Chinese society, they may result from other conflicts as well. It is entirely possible that many of Ms. Chen's persecutors were motivated by perceived social pressure, while secretly wishing that some of the "vulgar" calendars and magazines available in cities could be found in their little town. One cannot say how many of the Chinese people are simply afraid to admit to their appreciation of physical beauty, but the following account is suggestive. This is the experience of a highly educated and cultured Chinese psychiatrist who came to the United States in 1980:

> Shortly after my arrival in America, even the very first day, I noticed that the concept of sex in this country is very different, much

more liberal, than in China. While I was in the car going from Los Angeles to Long Beach where I would be living in the U.S., I was attracted by the huge, well-designed advertisements along the freeway. Once in a while a big picture of an almost nude girl shows up, seducing the drivers. I was shocked by their nudity, with only a limited part of the body covered. These pictures would be attractive to a normal, healthy man. When I first saw them I was seduced. I intended to enjoy it and watched carefully. And when I tried to do so, Confucius' teaching came to my mind: "You should not look at anything degenerating." I immediately took my glance away from it, staring directly ahead, holding my eyes fixed and pretending to have no interest in the picture of the nude girl. However, when the ad was almost behind me I could not keep from glancing back at it. (Liu Zhong-yi, 1987)

Restriction of Sexually Oriented Social Activities

For most of the history of the People's Republic of China, there have been severe restrictions on any social activity which includes or implies sexual expression of any kind. Plays and films which the government considers "obscene" cannot be shown anywhere. Chinese filmmakers are not permitted to include nude scenes, and such scenes are cut from foreign films before they are distributed. Even some songs are banned because they are "lustful." There is a well-known Taiwanese singer, Miss Deng Lijun, whose work is quite popular among mainland Chinese. The government's reaction to her is an excellent indicator of the general political climate. Her songs are allowed to circulate in mainland China at times when there is more personal freedom; whenever the political climate cools, it is forbidden to play Ms. Deng's music, and the media publish attacks on her work.

Until the comparative liberalization in the 1980s, there was no public nightlife in cities and towns—all theaters and cinemas closed before midnight, usually before 11:00 P.M. There were no nightclubs or cafes where young men and women could gather informally.

Personal adornment was also frowned upon. There were no beauty shops, and women did not use cosmetics because to do so was to risk being scolded. Almost from the founding of the People's Republic of China until the 1980s, women had dressed just like men, wearing the same colors and styles, unless they were willing to be labeled "hooligans." These restrictions are meant not only to prevent displays of luxury or individualistic expression, but to deemphasize sexual differences, as we can see from what Dr. Liu Zhongyi (1987) had to say about the differences between Chinese and American styles:

For most [American] women, even though they may not wear any nude-type of clothes [here the author seems to mean clothes revealing bare skin], as the clothes are so tight, the contour of the female body, with high breasts and thighs, is very clear; you can even see the buttock crease on the lower part of the back and the inguinal crease on the lower part of the abdomen. I am quite sure if my mom were still alive and saw women wearing this type of dress, she would scold them as "hoodlums without a sense of shame!" If they were blown up by a hurricane to any part of China, I am sure they would definitely be immediately surrounded by a crowd of people who would look at them disdainfully and with great curiosity.

There is hardly any opportunity for social contact between young men and women, especially outside the large towns which have dance halls (about which more will be said). In many high schools, girls and boys cannot sit together, and a girl who initiates a conversation with a boy is criticized as "shameless."

The censorious atmosphere leads to many personal injustices, like that described in a letter to *Jiefang Ri bao*, a Shanghai daily newspaper published by the government and reprinted in the overseas edition of the *People's Daily* of June 15, 1986. In her letter, a 20-year-old girl from Hunan province wrote that some years before, as a high school student, she had borrowed a mathematics exercise book from a male classmate. When she returned the book, she enclosed a note that said, "Your math is so good, I would like to learn from you in the future." When her teacher and classmates found out about the note, they turned against her, sneering and calling her "shameless." Even after she graduated from high school and began working in a factory, her coworkers avoided her. Her letter to the newspaper was the only possible outlet for her pain and indignation. While it is clear that there are elements of traditional conservatism at work in such incidents, it is also true that government policies, far from encouraging modernization, work to strengthen and deepen already entrenched attitudes. Policies motivated by the leaders' own sexual conservatism, and their desire to maintain strict social control, are also driven by hostility and suspicion toward the students and intellectuals who support more progressive policies.

One of the few exceptions to the social segregation of the sexes has been the occasional opportunity to meet at dance halls or institutionally sponsored dances. The Communist Party's policy on social dancing has been ambivalent at best. In 1953, the government ordered the closing of dance halls, and the women who worked there were given the same options as prostitutes—becoming actresses, workers, or peasants (Chou, 1971). Since then, dancing has been forbidden more often than not, with the decision depending on the prevailing political climate. In 1956, after an important political leader advocated dancing, dances were held every weekend all over the country under the sponsorship of colleges, universities, factories, and other institutions. Just a few months later, at the order of another, more highly placed official, the whole country stopped dancing. Similar revivals and suppressions of dancing accompanied subsequent changes in the political situation.

The most recent announcement giving permission for dancing, and even for commercial dance halls, was made by the central government in May of 1987. Then in early 1988, the Minister of Culture, the noted author Wang Mong, announced that, since no untoward incidents had occurred in more than six months since the reopening of the dance halls, dancing would be allowed to continue (*Centre Daily News*, January 4, 1988).

The decision to reopen the dance halls has been popular, especially among the youth. The number of halls has grown at a phenomenal rate. For example, an article published in the *Central Daily News* on April 26, 1988, reported that 112 dance halls had opened in Fujian province. Thirty of these were in Fuzhou, the provincial capital of the province, and about 3,000 people used these facilities every night. In Xiamen (Amoy) city, the famous special economic area of the province, 21 dance halls had opened (compared to only three during the Republican era). In 1987, more than 500,000 dance tickets were sold in Xiamen, though they were expensive—at 2–3 yuan, a single ticket cost 2–3% of the average monthly salary.

Devaluation of the Marriage Relationship

Humana and Wu (1982), describing the People's Republic of China as an "antierotic" society, point out that "the sexual side of marriage, extramarital relations and romantic feelings between Yin and Yang are either ignored, discouraged or prohibited." Although marriage is the only legal, officially accepted context for sexual expression, the needs of married couples are neglected. Many married couples are forced to live apart for anywhere from one to ten years, and sometimes even longer. According to official statistics, approximately 360,000 married persons live apart from their spouses, and this figure increases at a rate of 100,000 per year (*Centre Daily News*, September 18, 1989). Most of these separations occur because individual citizens are not free to move from one place to another or to change their places of employment. Where a person lives and works is determined by the government, which may assign a husband to work in one city and a wife to work in another. It is expected that the separated partners will "submit individual interests to Party and state interests." Most couples are allowed to reunite only once a year for about 14 days. The government pays for travel costs, which in 1989 amounted to 2.2 billion yuan (at that time, about U.S. $6 million). Anyone who applies for a change of employment in order to join his or her spouse may be required to pay for the privilege, in an amount ranging from thousands to tens of thousands of yuan—the equivalent to ten years' total earnings for the average worker (*Centre Daily News*, September 18, 1989).

Such separations, the general atmosphere of disregard for the needs of married couples, and the lack of adequate sex education (to be discussed) all contribute to marital dissatisfaction. Some estimate that as many as 60% of the Chinese are unhappy with their marriages (Burton, 1988), and the divorce rate is rising accordingly. The increasing divorce rate is a complex phenomenon. The influence of Western ideas of romantic love, women's increasing independence, and increased popular acceptance of extramarital affairs are also thought to be factors. Although couples seeking divorce are required to receive mediation, more than half a million couples divorce yearly.

Sex Crimes

In mainland China, a new word has been coined to label sexual behaviors which are illegal or officially held to be immoral. "Xingzuicuo" is compounded of three words—"xing," meaning "sex" or "sexual"; "zui," meaning crime; and "cuo," meaning "erroneous," "fault," "demerit," "wrong," or "mistaken." Thus "xingzuicuo" means either "sex crimes" or "sexual misconduct," depending on context.

The current perception in China is that both sex crimes (such as rape) and sexual misconduct (such as premarital and extramarital intercourse) have reached crisis proportions. Despite the official policy of suppressing sexual expression and severely punishing sex crimes, the crime rate continues to rise yearly. The government shows little awareness of the contribution its own puritanical policies have contributed to these problems. Instead, it attempts unsuccessfully to quell misbehavior by imposing increasingly harsh penalties.

It is difficult to assess the true extent of the apparent crisis, since "crime" and "misconduct" are not always clearly distinguished. Rape, pedophilia, and any behavior which "subjects women to indignities or carries out other gangster activities" are all clearly illegal, according to Articles 139 and 160 of the 1980 Criminal Law of the People's Republic of China. Prostitution may be treated as a sex crime or as sexual misconduct, depending upon the conditions; however, Article 140 of the

Criminal Law states that it is illegal "to force a female to engage in prostitution." The concept of "sexual misconduct" also includes premarital sex, extramarital sex, unmarried cohabitation, group sex, homosexual behavior, and other variant sexual behaviors.

Rape

The Chinese government does not publicize sex crime statistics, but some figures are available in academic journals. According to one researcher (Liu, 1987), the incidence of rape increased nationally 345% from 1979 to 1983; this trend was closely paralleled in Shanghai, China's most populous city, where rape incidence increased 377% in the same period.

Liu (1987) also found a significant increase in rape by teenagers; his findings are summarized in Table 9–1.

Juvenile Sexual Delinquents

The juvenile crime rate from 1979 to 1981 increased more than 25%, and "sex crimes" contributed significantly to this growth. According to statistics collected in three cities from 1980 to 1983, 13% of juvenile crimes were sex crimes, most committed by children between 13 and 15 years old. In the same period, in the Shanghai Juvenile Delinquent Correction Institution, 40% of the male inmates were charged with sexual crime or misconduct and 95% of the female inmates were charged with sexual misbehavior; some of these children were only 12 years old (H.X. Yang, 1988). The high proportion of sex offenders among female inmates suggests that incarceration is used not only to punish serious crimes, but also as a method of social control. In a later survey conducted over a three-month period and reported in the *Centre Daily News* (November 23, 1988), of 131 admissions to the Shanghai Juvenile Delinquent Correction Institution, 36% were sexual offenders.

Table 9–1. Increase in Incidence of Teenage Rape[a]

Year	Percentage
1980	(base year)
1981	150
1982	192
1983	311
1984	[b]
1985	142.5 of 1984 rate

[a]Based on Liu, Dalin, 1987.
[b]A slight decline in percentage, though absolute numbers increased.

Extramarital Sex

Extramarital affairs seem to be rather common in China, though they are conducted in such secrecy that little statistical information is available. Perhaps the best evidence of these affairs is divorce rates; Wu (1988) found that one-third of the divorces in Beijing from 1984 to 1985 were caused by extramarital relationships; if this finding is at all typical, then the increasing divorce rate must reflect an increase in the number of extramarital relationships. In one of the few surveys that has been done, Professor Pan at Chinese People's University in Beijing found that members of at least 10% of his sample of 600 couples had had extramarital sex (*Sing Tao Evening News*, September 24, 1988). Perhaps most significant is the latest finding in a nationwide survey (cited in Burton, 1990) that 69% of the people surveyed did not think extramarital affairs were wrong.

Hypocrisy and Resistance

As public attitudes increasingly diverge from official policies regarding sexual behavior, resistance is stiffened by popular awareness of hypocrisy on the part of government officials. Especially since the Cultural Revolution, disclosures about the private lives of Chinese leaders have undermined their credibility as moral exemplars. Not only is political corruption widespread, but it has become obvious that far from being puritanical, many leaders were nothing less than libertines. For example, Ye Zhiqiu, an expert on the history of the Chinese Communist Party, has reported that former Premier Chou acted as a procurer for Party Chairman Mao Tsedong. On one occasion in 1964, Chou organized a singing and dancing group under the leadership of the General Political Department of the Chinese People's Liberation Army. The group consisted of eighteen young girls who were told that their task was a secret. One girl at a time was sent to Mao's room to "perform"—in fact, to provide their country's most revered leader with sexual companionship (*Centre Daily News*, January 8, 1990).

Knowing that their leaders do not themselves respect the limits they set for others, ordinary people often simply do what they wish, albeit secretly. It is clear that the Communist regime has been no more effective than the Ming and Ching emperors in exterminating basic sexual instincts. This does not mean, however, that repressive policies have been without effect. One particularly unfortunate result has been such pervasive ignorance about human sexuality that even those who are bold enough to seek sexual satisfaction have little idea how to approach their goal.

SEX OBSCURANTISM AND SEX EDUCATION

The Need for Sex Education

In line with its general policy of suppressing any discussion of sexuality, the Chinese government neglected the development of sex education courses for the general curriculum. It was not until the early 1980s that model programs were developed, and even then, discussion was usually limited to the necessity of using contraception to limit population growth. In his book *China: Alive in the Bitter Sea*, Fox Butterfield (1982) gave a vivid example of the impact that enforced ignorance has on people's personal lives. Describing an interview with a highly educated intellectual, he wrote:

> When I asked if she had ever experienced an orgasm, Hua's face furrowed into a frown.... "What is that?" she asked in reply. She had never had any such sensation. Intercourse, as she knew it, consumed three or four minutes and ended when her husband withdrew. The only position they had tried, she said, was for her to lie flat on her back and her husband to climb on top of her. Had she ever tried oral sex then? I asked. "What is that, kissing?" she responded.

The few statistics that have been gathered indicate that such ignorance is not uncommon. For example, Pan (cited in Burton, 1990) found that men reached orgasm 70% of the time, women only 40% of the time. The data also remove any doubt that education would be helpful. Liu's finding that 60% of urban married couples surveyed have experimented with various sexual positions and Pan's finding that 6% of the heterosexual couples he surveyed had had anal intercourse at least once suggest that people would be open to new information about their partners' needs. It is significant that Liu found experimentation among *urban* couples; the situation in the countryside is quite different. Thirty-four percent of rural couples (compared to 17% of urban couples) said they engaged in less than a minute of foreplay—sometimes none at all. Not surprisingly, 37% of rural wives described intercourse as painful (Burton, 1990). In light of Western findings that sexual satisfaction is positively correlated to level of education, the urban-rural split in Chinese sexual behaviors underlines the need for sex education, all the more because, while urban couples may be more adventurous sexually, they are not necessarily more satisfied. Professor Pan's sample of 600 couples were all residents of big cities, and 70% of them said they were unhappy with their sex lives (*Sing Tao Evening News*, September 24, 1988); a random

survey of married couples living in Shanghai found that 45% were unhappy with their sexual relationships.

Obscurantism: Sex Education Policies and Publications from 1949 to 1980

The only major political leader to advocate the need for sex education was Premier Chou En-lai. In 1963, he invited about a dozen famous
medical professors to meet with him to discuss the issue. He expressed
his belief that teenagers should receive instruction before girls reach the
age of menarche and boys begin to experience nocturnal emissions. He
recalled that when he was an adolescent attending Nan-kai High School
in Tientsin, he was given lessons on human sexuality that remained useful throughout his life. He argued that courses in human sexuality should
be coeducational, so that the subject would seem less forbidden and mysterious (Ye Gongshao, 1983).

Unfortunately, Party Chairman Mao's emphasis on class struggle
had a destructive effect on any attempt to develop sex education curric-
ula. Premier Chou, who had been diagnosed with cancer in 1972, was
well aware that he was the only person in a position to express openly
and directly the need for such programs, and made every effort to speak
out before his death. When Chou was hospitalized in April 1973, the
director of his medical team was Professor Wu Jieping, then the vice
president of the Chinese Academy of Medical Sciences. When Professor
Wu visited the Premier on April 12, they discussed sex education again
(Wu Jieping, 1980). In 1975, when his illness was clearly terminal, Chou
made a point of meeting with medical educators and public health officers to encourage them to develop thorough and accurate sex education
programs. When Premier Chou died on January 8, 1976, at age 78, a
valuable advocate of sexual enlightenment was lost, but his influence
did continue to have an effect.

At the time of Chou's death, not only was there a complete lack of
systematic sex education, but only few sex booklets had been published.
Sex Knowledge (Xing-zhi-shi), published in 1956, was the first modern
book on sexuality that had not been translated from a European language. The editor, Yu Guangyuan, a famous dermatologist practicing in
Shanghai, collected eighteen articles that had been written by himself
and others, for a special sexuality issue of *Popular Medicine* (Dazong
Yixue), a popular medical magazine with wide circulation. Another much
more famous Chinese sex education booklet, *Knowledge of Sex* (Xing-di-
zhi-shi), was published in 1957. This booklet represented the primary

effort to provide some sexual information to the Chinese people. The authors were three physicians: Wen-bin Wang and Zhi-yi Zhao, both gynecologists, and Ming-xin Tan, a neurologist. All three worked in the most prestigious hospital in China, Beijing United Hospital. Most of the booklet is devoted to social topics, such as love and marriage, and medical topics, such as sexual dysfunctions. Only a few pages discuss such aspects of sexual relationships as arousal, sexual responses, and frequency of intercourse. Yet, for more than twenty years, *Knowledge of Sex* was virtually the only sex booklet available to a population of 800 to 900 million people! Several million copies were printed and sold.

During the Cultural Revolution (June 1966–October 1976), any discussion or activity relating to sex was decried as "bourgeois," "lustful," and "decadent." Proposals for sex education were condemned as resulting from the corrosive influence of bourgeois ideas. Needless to say, the publishers and authors of *Knowledge of Sex* were criticized and attacked by the Red Guards and "revolutionary masses."

A single incident illustrates the strength of the resistance to instituting sex education. In 1972, Professor Ye Gongshao was invited to be one of the editors of the junior high school textbook *Physiology and Hygiene*. Ye, who has an excellent reputation as a leading scholar in the field of adolescent hygiene and a well-known social activist, wrote a chapter on "Reproductive Organs." Half of the people attending a meeting to finalize the text opposed the inclusion of this material! Only after Professor Ye mentioned that it was Premier Chou who had asked her to write the chapter did her opponents agree to adopt it.

A New Enlightenment: Sex Education Publications and Programs after 1980

In 1980, heartened by the end of the Cultural Revolution and inspired by the memory of Chou En-lai's support, a few authors and publishers began to produce new materials. The first effort was a new edition of *Knowledge of Sex* published by People's Medical Publishing House. (This edition is referred to as *Sex Knowledge* in Butterfield, 1982, and Weisskopf, 1980.) Two of the book's authors had died. The surviving author, Professor Tan Ming-xin, revised the text that had earned so much condemnation for him and his coauthors. He deleted any language which seemed too explicit, and the resulting text, consisting of only 54,000 Chinese characters, was only 74 pages long. Also, Professor Tan adopted a more conservative tone generally. The legacy of fear created by the Cultural Revolution explains why Weisskopf (1980) could accurately describe the book as "old-fashioned by Western standards." Butterworth (1982) comments, "...the only sex manual I ever saw in China took an even stricter view of the need to limit the frequency of intercourse... [recommending a] normal routine of 'once every week or two.'" Nonetheless, the first edition of 2.5 million copies, released in June, 1980, was sold out almost immediately, and some people resold their copies at nearly double the original price.

By August of 1980, there had been four reprintings of the new edition of *Knowledge of Sex*, totaling 2.3 million copies. From 1980 to 1984, more than ten new sex handbooks were published. Two of them became best-sellers. Both were written by two gynecologists, Drs. Han Xiangyang and Lang Jinghuo. The first, *Required Readings in Wedding Hygiene* was originally published in September 1980, and by November 1981 had already been reprinted eight times, for a total of more than 7.5 million copies. The second, *Questions and Answers about Wedding Hygiene*, published in July 1984, was first printed in a large edition of 4.2 million copies.

Finally, in the mid-1980s, a number of pressures led national and local officials to acknowledge the need for sex education programs:

1. Since early in the decade, several leading experts had been pressing for the establishment of such programs. Three people in particular were most influential, thanks to their high social positions and excellent reputations: Professor Wu Jieping, whose special relationship with Premier Chou was described above; Professor Ye Gongshao, the expert on adolescent health mentioned above; and Dr. Zhou Jianren, a former professor who was then vice chair of the Standing Committee Members of the National People's Congress. (Zhou Jianren was the brother of Zhou Shuren, one of China's greatest modern writers, who used the pen name Lu Hsun.) As early as 1928, Zhou Jianren had written a book titled *Sex Education*. Wu, Ye, and Zhou's numerous articles explaining the need for sex education were widely published in the popular press.

2. Population growth continued to be a very serious problem. A birth control program had been instituted in January 1973, but it became unavoidably clear that to implement the program effectively, young people would have to be given sexual information essential to understanding and using contraception.

3. Rates of teenage pregnancy, juvenile sex crime, and sexually transmitted diseases seemed to be increasing (see above). It was argued that sex education offered the best hope for diminishing these problems (Wu Jieping, 1987).

4. Finally, as a result of the new "open-door" policy of receptiveness to Western cultural influence, and a simultaneous increase in personal freedoms, the Chinese people were expressing a desire to improve their lives, including their sexual lives (for more information, see the next section, "Human Rights and Sexual Liberation"). It was against this background that researchers gathered the data on sexual dissatisfaction just noted. In addition, medical professionals felt that the numbers of patients they were treating for sexual dysfunction demonstrated a need for improved education. According to Professor Kang Jin, president of the Shanghai Committee of Rehabilitation of Male Dysfunctions, in 1989 at least 20% of China's adult male population were suffering from some type of sexual dysfunction (*World Journal*, August 22, 1989).

The first high school sex education courses were introduced in 1981 in Shanghai. As noted earlier, sex education in China has always been related to the need for population control and contraception (Fraser, 1978, 1983), but the new courses had a broader scope. The city of Shanghai has led in promoting high school sex education, and the following account of Shanghai's programs gives a good picture of developments in China from 1986.

In early 1986, 40 Shanghai middle schools, about 10% of the city's total, introduced an experimental sex education course for mixed classes in the 12–13 age group. In addition to helping students understand the physiological and psychological changes they were undergoing, the course was designed to teach hygiene and sexual morality. Those introducing the course noted that according to medical surveys over 60% of the girls in the 12–13 age group have started menstruation and puberty in boys now begins at an age of 14.1 years. Both educators and officials attribute the general lack of attention to sex education in the schools to the legacy of feudalism that has dominated China for thousands of years ("News Briefs," *China Reconstructs* [North American Edition], 35: 63–64, 1986).

These experiments in sex education were so successful that six months later, on June 7, 1986, nearly 100 Shanghai middle schools gave sex education courses. And, by February 1988, 6,000 middle schools all over China had instituted sex education courses. Thirteen of the 28 provinces, including Shanghai, Jiangsu, Tianjin, and Helongjiang, had made sex education courses part of the standard middle school curriculum. The State Council announced that sex education courses would soon be established in middle schools nationwide (*Centre Daily News*, February 23, 1988).

On May 23, 1988, the country's first college-level sexology course was introduced at China People's University in Beijing. This special two-week program, called "Training Workshop on Sex Science," consisted of workshops on 20 topics conducted by 17 professors and experts. The program was attended by 120 people from 26 of China's 28 provinces (*Centre Daily News,* May 26, 1988).

The latter half of the 1980s was a time of tension between the acknowledged need for sex education and continued pressure within the government to maintain tight social control. Thus in 1985 the government limited the printing of an updated *Handbook of Sex Knowledge,* and in 1986 it ruled that only two publishing houses would be permitted to publish books on sex; yet in 1988 it allowed the showing of a film which explicitly referred to the *Handbook.* The movie, entitled "Mandarin Duck Apartments" (to the Chinese, a pair of mandarin ducks symbolize an affectionate couple), includes a scene in which an old woman counsels a newlywed who feels that sex is dirty and shameful. The old woman shows her the *Handbook,* explaining that findings in sexual science show that women have as much right as men to enjoy sex.

While school-based programs were of great importance, public discussion of sexuality was so new and so essential that much of the work that needed to be done was in the areas of professional development and general adult education. The author of this book, as a pioneer in the discipline of sexology, was responsible for much of the work in these fields, and a brief review of this work will complete the picture of progress made in the 1980s:

1. To fill the need for distributing basic sex information as widely as possible, 84 articles by the author were published in 15 magazines and 7 newspapers, including the most popular magazines in China, such as *Reader's Digest* (distributing several million copies per issue), *China Youth* (distributing more than 3 million copies per issue), *Popular Medicine* (more than 1 million copies per issue), and *Health* (more than 1 million copies per issue).

2. The author's special series of columns entitled "Essays on Sex Education" was published in *Required Readings for Parents,* the leading national monthly magazine on child and adolescent education. The series consisted of ten rather long articles on various aspects of sexuality and sex education, published from January to October 1985. It was the first systematic treatment of such topics to be published since the founding of the People's Republic of China in 1949. Besides providing adult education, the articles served to enhance school-based programs by giving parents and educators information needed for child guidance. To further the goals of

providing all Chinese with a common base of sexual knowledge and creating a sound foundation for sex education policy, the magazine's publisher (Beijing Publishing House) sent a copy of each issue to each member of the Political Bureau of the Central Committee of the Chinese Communist Party. The titles of the individual articles suggest the range of comprehensive, fundamental information included:

1. Why Is Sex Education Necessary?
2. A Survey of Sex Education in Other Countries
3. Sex, Gender, and Sex Role
4. The Moral, Intellectual, Physical, and Aesthetic Aspects of Sex Education
5. Sex Education for Children
6. Sex Education for Adolescents
7. Sex Education for Young Adults
8. On Masturbation
9. Sex Education in the Family, in School, and in Society
10. Lu Hsun (Zhou Shuren) and his brothers Zhou Cuo-ren and Zhou Jianren on sex education.

3. From July 22 to August 7, 1985, the First National Workshop on Sex Education was held in Shanghai. This was the first such conference convened in mainland China since 1949. It was an interdisciplinary workshop, attended by more than 80 professionals from 18 provinces, most of them in the fields of birth control, sociology, urology, and high school and college education.

As a pioneer in the new interdisciplinary field of sexology, the author was the major instructor, delivering eight lectures and an address concerning the need to found a national society for sex education. During the workshop, the preparatory committee of the Chinese Sex Education Research Society was organized. (This workshop was reported in more than 14 newspapers published in China, Hong Kong, Singapore, the United States, and France.)

4. In 1985 the author served both as chief editor and as a major contributor for the compilation of an updated *Handbook of Sex Knowledge* (see References for details). Although it was intentionally the most up-to-date text of its kind, the book could not, of course, include any descriptions of sexual positions or any nude illustrations (except anatomical drawings). Despite these self-imposed restrictions, the first printing was limited to 500,000 copies by a decision of the Central Publishing Bureau.

HUMAN RIGHTS AND SEXUAL LIBERATION

No discussion of changing sexual attitudes in China can be complete without a description of the broader political context. As we have discussed in detail, progress in modernizing sexual relationships and education has frequently been hampered by a generally repressive political atmosphere. Conversely, any possibility of significant sexual liberation is intimately (if not always explicitly) related to the broader struggle for increased political and personal freedom.

In the late 1970s there was a spontaneous mass movement for democracy. The roots of this development may be found in the "April Fifth Movement" of 1976. After Chou En-lai's death in January of 1976, the Gang of Four (heads of the new government) had forbidden any public mourning, but on the annual day of mourning, April 5 (traditionally known as Qing Ming Jie, or the "Pure Brightness Festival"), nothing could prevent a great crowd of hundreds of thousands from gathering around the Martyrs' Memorial in Beijing's Tiananmen Square to express their affection for the dead premier (Tiananmen means "Gate of Heavenly Peace"). This became known as the April Fifth incident, and was seen as historically parallel to the demonstration on May 4, 1919, when 3,000 Peking students from 13 institutions gathered in front of the Gate of Heavenly Peace and ushered in the May Fourth Movement. The April 5 demonstration, organized by the opposition to the Gang of Four, represented a pervasive disillusionment at the popular level. Maurice Meisner (1986) describes these events vividly:

> ...People came in increasing numbers over a period of four days, not only with wreaths but also with poems, wall posters, and speeches eulogizing Chou [Zhou] En-lai, and in many making veiled criticisms of the "Gang of Four"...but several thousand who remained at nightfall were attacked by the urban militia. Some were wounded, many arrested, and several hundred imprisoned.
>
> The "April Fifth Movement," as it soon came to be called, became a powerful political symbol over the years to come—symbolic of the spirit of popular resistance to a despotic state. (Meisner, 1986, pp. 424–425)

From then on, the phrase "April Fifth Youth" was used to refer to young people who struggle for democracy and freedom.

The next major move toward democracy was the "Democracy Wall" movement of 1978 and 1979. During this brief period, the government allowed young people to express their desire for personal freedom and democracy by placing "big character" posters on a wall that came to be known as "Democracy Wall." Roger Garside, an eyewitness who spent hundreds of hours at Democracy Wall during the time that young Chinese were freely speaking their minds there, described it in detail in more than 30 pages of his *Coming Alive: China After Mao* (1981):

> It is an unimpressive stretch of wall about two hundred yards long and twelve feet high....For four months in the winter of 1978–1979 voices came from that wall which were heard around the world and earned it the name Democracy Wall....

Some of these posters actually criticized the late leader Mao Tsedong by name. One poster titled "The Fifth Modernization—Democracy," whose author Wei Jing-sheng was eventually sentenced to fifteen years in jail, said, "The people have finally learned where their goal is. They have a clear orientation and a real leader—the democratic banner" (Garside, 1981).

The Democracy Wall was also used for advocating sexual liberation. The author vividly recalls visiting the wall on February 20, 1979, and seeing two poems about sex written by "Sasa" and "Manman" (two common women's names which were probably pseudonyms). One was titled "The Eulogy of Sexual Desire," the other "Open Sex." The entire text of the second poem is translated below. The phrases which are in brackets in this translation were originally written in English (which was very unusual on "Democracy Wall"), though word order has been corrected from "sex open" to "open sex."

Xing (sex) Kaifang (open) [Open Sex]

Friend, are you an April Fifth youth?
Let us stand together to advocate open sex.
Oh, you are studying English,
Good, please remember this new phrase:
[Open sex.]

1979, it will be Open Sex Year,
If we take a figure of speech:
This year is a girl,
"Open sex" is the little wool hat on her head,
If you do not put it on,
You are not modern at all.

Open sex,
Open sex,
Sweep away all of the feudal ideology.

Open sex,
Open sex,
Advocate the modernization of life-style.

Open sex, [O.K.]
[Nudity, O.K.]

By March 5, 1979, these poems had already been scrubbed away. On the remaining fragments of the posters criticisms such as "no pornography" had been scrawled. In posters like these, China's youth first made a courageous stand on the importance of sexual openness to their country's modernization.

During the nationwide demonstration by university students in the winter of 1986–1987, there were also some posters advocating sexual freedom. That demonstration led to a crackdown in the ranks of the Chinese Communist Party, and the expulsion of three very famous intellectuals: the astrophysicist Fang Lizhi, a leading Chinese dissident; Liu Binyan, a leading journalist and writer; and Wang Ruowang, an elderly author.

Meanwhile, the government's ambivalence regarding the new programs in sex education was increasing. It was all too tempting to conclude that such problems as the spread of sexually transmitted diseases were simply the result of increased sexual openness. Thus it is not surprising that, after the demonstrations at Tiananmen Square in 1989, the government fell into its old habit of including sexual restrictions in a wave of political repression. The most recent sign of a resurgence of repression came in July 1990, when the vice president of the Supreme People's Court, Lin Zhun, issued a new decree instituting the death penalty for traffickers in prostitution and/or pornography (*Sing Pao Daily News*, July 18, 1990).

But the latest wave of repression is certainly not the end of the story. While sexual liberation was not a major explicit goal of the 1989 democracy movement, its importance was understood and its value implicit in one of the loveliest events that occurred then. During the hunger strike in Tiananmen Square, a wedding was held for one of the leaders of the demonstrators. The bride and groom, the maid of honor (the General Commander Chai Ling, now an internationally known heroine of the struggle for democracy) and the best man (Chai's husband, the Vice General Commander Feng Congde) were all fasting, as were the classmates attending the wedding. Yet all the celebrants were laughing joyously (*World Journal*, April 4, 1990). The wedding was the ideal symbol of the connection between the longing for liberty and the desire for love, marriage, and personal happiness.

As the tide of modernization overtakes China, sexual freedom will certainly have its place among the vital human rights the people will enjoy in the future.

Notes on Romanization

It is a difficult task to romanize the Chinese names and terms that are used in this book. Although it seems best to use the pinyin system, which has been adopted nationwide in mainland China as the official standard way to spell Chinese characters, one has to bear in mind that in the West much of the general public is familiar with spellings adopted from other systems. The only alternative seems to be to use the pinyin system for all Chinese proper names (including names of historical dynasties and various publications) except in those cases in which a different spelling seems more likely to be recognized. In direct quotations, of course, the spelling originally used is kept unchanged.

Regardless of how a name is romanized, the text follows the Chinese rule by which the family name precedes given names—for example, Ruan Fang Fu rather than Fang Fu Ruan. Even within these rules, a name spelled with the pinyin system might be written in a number of ways. For example, the author's name might appear in a number of forms, including all those shown below, all of which are equivalent:

Fang Fu Ruan	Fang F. Ruan	Fangfu Ruan
Fang-fu Ruan	Fang-Fu Ruan	Ruan Fangfu
Ruan, Fang Fu	Ruan Fang-fu	Ruan Fang-Fu

In some instances, Westerners do follow the Chinese rule of writing the family name first. For example, Westerners write "Mao Tse-tung," and not "Tse-tung Mao," and "Deng Xiaoping," rather than "Xiaoping Deng." In this book, the rule will be followed in most cases.

Since different persons prefer different ways of writing the same name, sometimes alternative spellings are listed parenthetically. This should be helpful to readers who are familiar with some Chinese proper names from older translations, and might be surprised to meet "Confucius, Tao, Taoist, Lu Hsun, Li Po, Peking, and Canton" in the guise of "Kongzi, Dao, Daoist, Lu Xun, Li Bo, Beijing, and Guangzhou." The following list includes many Chinese proper names which have already been translated in Western literature using the Wade-Giles System or other systems.

Pinyin System	Wade-Giles or Other Systems
Anhui	Anhwei
Beijing	Peking
Chen Yun	Ch'en Yun*
Chengdu	Chengtu
Chongqing	Chungking
Cixi (Dowager Empress)	Tz'u Hsi
Dalian	Dairen, Talien
Daode Jing	Tao-te-ching
Daojia	Tao-chia
Daojiao	Tao-chiao
Daozang (Taoist Canon)	Tao Tsang
Deng Xixian	Teng Hsi-hsien
Deng Xiaoping (1904–)	Teng Hsiao-p'ing
Deng Yingchao (1903–)	Teng Ying-ch'ao
Duan Xiu Pian	Tuan-hsiu-pien
Fang zhong	Fang chung
Fujian	Fukien
Fuxi	Fu Hsi
Fuzhou	Foochow
Gansu	Kansu
Gaozi	Kao-tzu
Ge Hong (A.D. 281–341)	Ko Hung, Pao Po Tzu
Guan Zhong (?–645 B.C.)	Kuang Chung, Kuan I-wu
Guangdong	Kwangtung
Guangzhou	Canton, Kwangchow
Guangxi Zhuangzu Zizhiqu	Kwangsi Chuang Aut. Reg.
Guilin	Kweilin
Guiyang	Kweiyang
Guizhou	Kweichow
Guo Moruo (1892–1978)	Kuo Mo-jo
Guomindang	Kuomintang
Hangzhou	Hangchow, Hang-chau
Hebei	Hepei
Heilongjiang	Heilungkiang

*In the Wade-Giles system the apostrophe (') is used to indicate the pronunciation.

Henan	Honan, Hunan
Hu Shi (1891–1962)	Hu Shih
Hu Yaobang (1915–1989)	Hu Yao-pang
Hua Guofeng (1921–)	Hua Kuo-feng
Huang He	Yellow River
Hubei	Hupei, Hupeh
Ji Yun (A.D. 1724–1805)	Chi Yun
Jiangsu	Kiangsu
Jiangxi	Kiangsi
Jilin	Kirin
Jin (A.D. 1115–1234)	Chin (Jurchen)
Jinan	Tsinan
Kangxi (reigned A.D. 1661–1722)	K'ang-hsi
Kongzi (551–497 B.C.)	K'ung-tzu, Confucius
Kongjiao	K'ung-chiao
Lanzhou	Lanchow
Laozi	Lao-tzu
Lu Dongbin (A.D. 789–?)	Lu Tung-pin
Lu Xun (1881–1936)	Lu Hsun
Mao Zedong (1893–Sept. 6, 1976)	Mao Tse-tung
Mengzi (313?–289 B.C.)	Meng-tzu, Mencius
Nanjing	Nanking
Nei Mogol Zizhiqu	Inner Mongolia Aut. Reg.
Ningxia Huizu Zizhiqu	Ningsia Hui Aut. Reg.
Pan Ku (A.D. 32–92)	Ban Gu
Qi	Ch'i
Qin (221–206 B.C.)	Ch'in
Qing (A.D. 1644–1912)	Ch'ing, Manchu
Qingdao	Tsingtao
Qinghai	Tsinghai
Rujia	Ju-chia
Ruan Fangfu	Juan, Fang-fu; Ruan, Fongfu
Shaanxi	Shensi
Shandong	Shantung
Shanxi	Shansi
Shaoxing	Shaohsing
Shen Nong	Shen Nung
Shengni Niehai	Seng-ni-nieh-hai
Sichuan	Szechuan
Song (A.D. 960–1279)	Sung
Sun Kaidi	Sun Kaiti
Suzhou	Soochow
Taibei	Taipei
Tang (A.D. 618–907)	T'ang
Tianjin	Tientsin

Wang Chongyang (A.D. 1112–1170)	Wang Chung-yang
Wen Yidao	Wen I-to
Xia (about 21st–16th B.C.)	Hsia
Xi'an	Sian
Xiang Yan Cong Shu	Hsiang-yen-ts'ung-shu
Xinjiang Uygur Zizhiqu	Sinkiang Uighur Aut. Reg.
Xizang Zizhiqu	Tibet Aut. Reg.
Xun (about 22nd B.C.)	Shun
Yan'an	Yenan
Yi Jing	*I-Ching* (*Book of Changes*)
Yi Xin Fang	I-hsin-fang
Yuewei Caotang Biji (A.D. 1800)	Yueh Wei Tsao-Tung Pi-Chi
Zhang Baiduan [Ziyang Zhenren]	Chang Po-Tuan
(A.D. 984–1082)	
Zhao Ziyang (1919–)	Chao Tzu-yang
Zhejiang	Chekiang
Zhengzhou	Chengchow
Zhongguo Qingnian (Chinese Youth)	Chung-kuo Ch'ing-nien
Zhou (1111–249 B.C.)	Chou
Zhou Enlai (1898–Jan. 8, 1976)	Chou En-lai
Zhou Erfu (1914–)	Chou Erh-fu
Zhou Jianren (1888–1984)	Chou Chien-jen
Zhou Shaoxian (1908–)	Chou Shao-hsien

References with Selected
Annotations

References in English are not specially noted. References in Chinese give a Romanization of the publication's original Chinese title, followed by the English translation(s) of the title (by the author of this book and/or by others) without any special notation that the original language is Chinese. For example:

A Chinese book

Hsuan Wei Hshin In (*Mental Images of the Mysteries and Subtleties of Sexual Techniques, or The Sacred Seal in the Heart*).

A Chinese article

"Annotated Notes on Talks on the Super Tao in the World: Seven Hurts and Eight Advantages." *Hunan Zhongyi Xueyuan Xuebao (Journal of Hunan Traditional Chinese Medical College)*. 1980(1): 27–32.

For references in languages other than English or Chinese, the title is given in English translation, followed by an italicized notation of the original language of publication. For example:

A History of Traditional Chinese Medicine: Herbs, Acupuncture, and Regimen. In Japanese.

Ban Gu (Ed.) [A.D. 32–92]. (1983).: *Han Su (History of the Han)*. Reprint, Beijing: Zhong-hua Books Co.

Beijing Public Security Bureau. (Ed.) (1988). *Beijing Fengbi Jiyuan Jishi (The reports on closings of brothels in Beijing)*. Beijing: China Peace Press.

Benjamin, H. (1966). *The transsexual phenomenon*. New York: Julian Press.

Beurdeley, M., et al. (1969). *The clouds and the rain*. London: Hammond and Hammond.

Blofeld, J. (1978). *Taoism: The road to immortality*. Reprint, 1985. Boston: Shambhala.

Bullough, V. L. (1976). *Sexual variance in society and history.* New York: Wiley.

Bullough, V., & Bullough, Bonnie. (1987). India and China: Other views. In *Women and prostitution: A social history.* (Revised Edition of *Prostitution: An illustrated social history,* published by Crown Publishers in 1978), pp. 81–109. Buffalo, NY: Prometheus Books.

Bullough, V. L., & Ruan, F. F. (1988). China's children. (Editorials). *The Nation* 246, 848–849.

Bullough, V. L., & Ruan, F. F. (1990). Sex education in Mainland China. *Health Education* 21(2): 16–19.

Burton, S. (1988). The sexual revolution hits China: Reform has brought a permissiveness that unsettles many. *Time* (September 12): 65.

Burton, S. (1990). Straight talk on sex in China. *Time* (May 14): 82.

Butterfield, F. (1980). Love and sex in China. *New York Times Magazine,* January 13, 1980.

Butterfield, F. (1982). *China: Alive in the bitter sea.* Chapter 6: Sex without joy: Love and marriage, pp. 129–161. New York: Times Books.

Chai, C., & Chai, W. (Trans. & Ed.) (1965). *A treasury of Chinese literature.* New York: Appleton-Century-Crofts.

Chan, Wing-tsit. (Trans. & comp.). (1963). *A source book in Chinese philosophy.* Princeton, NJ: Princeton University Press.

Chan, Wing-tsit. (1983). "Taoism." In *Encyclopaedia Americana,* Volume 26, pp. 276–277.

Chang, J. S. [1888–1970]. (Trans. H. S. Levy) (1967). *Sex histories: China's first modern treatise on sex education.* Yokohama, Japan: Po-yuan Press. [Also published, New York: Paragon Book Gallery.]

Chang, J. (1977). *The Tao of love and sex: The ancient Chinese way to ecstasy.* London: Wildwood House; New York: Dutton.

Chang, J. (1980). Understanding the Tao of loving. *British Journal of Sexual Medicine* 7(67): 36–41.

Chang, J. (1983). *The Tao of the loving couple: True liberation through the Tao.* New York: Dutton.

Chang, K. C. (1977). *The archaeology of ancient China,* 3rd ed. New Haven, CT: Yale University Press.

Chang, S. T. (1985). The Tao of sex wisdom. In *The Great Tao,* pp. 295–327. San Francisco: Tao Publishing.

Chang, S. T. (1986). *The Tao of sexology: The book of infinite wisdom.* San Francisco: Tao Publishing.

Chen, T. Y. (1928). *Zhongguo Funu Shenghuoshi (The story of the Chinese women).* Shanghai: Commercial Press, Ltd.

Chen Sen. (1849). *Ping-hua Bao Jan (A mirror of theatrical life).* The edition used for this book is an undated Ching Dynasty edition at the Beijing Library. There are a total of 20 volumes.

Chen Xiyi [A.D. ?–989]. (1986). *Fang Shu Hsuan Chi (The mysterious essence of bedchamber techniques).* Reprint in Tan Ching (Ed.)(1986). *Zhong-guo gu-yan xi-ping cong-kan (Chinese Classical Erotic Rare Book Series),* No. 13. Taipei, Taiwan: Tan-ch'ing Book Co.

Cheng, L., Furth, C., & Yip, H. M. (1984). *Women in China: Bibliography of available English language materials.* Berkeley: Institute of East Asia Studies, University of California at Berkeley.

Chia, Mantak, & Chia, Maneewan. (1986). *Healing love through the Tao: Cultivative female sexual energy.* Huntington, NY: Healing Tao Books.

Chi, M., & Winn, M. (1984). *Taoist secrets of love: Cultivating male sexual energy.* New York: Aurora Press.

Chou, E. (1971). *The dragon and the phoenix.* New York: Arbor House.

Cleary, T. (Trans.) (1987). *Understanding reality: A Taoist alchemical classic. With a concise commentary by Liu I-ming.* Honolulu: University of Hawaii Press. A translation of *Wu chen pien* by Chang Po-tuan; see Zhang Beiduan (1987).

Cohen, J. A. (1968). *The criminal process in the People's Republic of China 1949–1963: An introduction.* Cambridge, MA: Harvard University Press.

Crump, J. I., Jr. (Trans.) (1970). *Chan-kuo tse.* London: Oxford University Press. The original work was published during the third to first centuries B.C.

Day, C. B. (1978) *The philosophers of China: Classical and contemporary.* Secaucus, NJ: The Citadel Press.

DeWoskin, K. J. (Trans.) (1983). *Doctors, diviners, and magicians of ancient China.* Translations from the Oriental Classics (Ed. W. T. de Bary *et al.*). New York: Columbia University Press. Biographies translated from *History of the Later Han, Records of the Three Kingdoms,* and *History of Chin.*

Deng Xixian. (1598). *Hsiu Chen Yen I (A popular exposition of the methods of regenerating the primary vitalities).* Deng Xixian (Tzu Chin Juang Yao Ta Hsien, the Great Immortal of the Purple-gold Splendor), was a famous Ming dynasty Taoist monk. This is a handbook of Taoists' sexual techniques (physiological alchemy). The Chinese text used here was hand-copied from a Ming dynasty blockprint (A.D. 1598) in the Beijing Library Rare Books Division by Fang Fu Ruan, in 1985; another edition is Tan Ching. (Ed.) (1986). *Zhong-guo gu-yan xi-ping cong-kan (Chinese Classical Erotic Rare Book Series),* No. 29.

Douglas, N., & Slinger, P. (1979). *Sexual secrets: The alchemy of ecstasy.* New York: Destiny Books.

Douglas, N., & Slinger, P. (1981). *The pillow book: The erotic sentiment and the paintings of India, Nepal, China, and Japan.* New York: Destiny Books.

Du Jiaming, Yi Xiao, & Xiong Hong. (1988). *Jingti: Xingbin zhai Zhongguo manyan (Watch out for: STDs are spreading in China).* Beijing: Zhongguo Zoyue Zuban Gongsi.

Etiemble. (Trans. J. Hogarth) (1970). *Yun Yu: An essay on eroticism and love in ancient China.* Geneva: Nagel Publishers.

Fairbank, J. K. (1986). *The great Chinese revolution 1800–1985.* New York: Harper & Row.

Fan, Wenlan. (1965). *Zhongguo Tongshi Jianbian (A brief survey of Chinese history),* rev. ed., Vol. 3, Part 2. Beijing: People's Publishing House.

Fang Chun-ie. (Ed) (1982). *Law annual report of China 1982/3.* Hong Kong: Kingsway International Publications, Ltd.

Feng M. L. [A.D. 1574–1646]. (1981). *Hsin-Shih Heng-Yen (Stories to awaken men, or Lasting words to awaken the world).* (First ed., A.D. 1627) Reprint, Fuzhou: Fujian People's Publishing House.

Feng Yuanjun [1900–1974]. (Trans. Yang Xianyi, & Gladys) (1983). *An outline history of classical Chinese literature.* Hong Kong: Joint Publishing Co.

Franzblau, A. N., & Etiemble. (1977). *Erotic art of China: A unique collection of Chinese prints and poems devoted to the art of love.* New York: Crown Publishers.

Fraser, S. E. (1978). Sexual behavior and social education in China. *Journal of Sex Education and Therapy* 4 (1): 40–42.

Fraser, S. E. (1983). Sex education? Population education? A new school programme for China's adolescents. *British Journal of Sexual Medicine* (97): 27–32.

Friend, R. (1978). How does China treat homosexuals? *Eastern Horizon* July: 36–37.

Fu, Qinjia. (1975). *Zhongkuo Daojiao Shi (A history of Taoism in China),* 5th ed. Taipei: Taiwan Commercial Press.

Gao Anming. (1989). China's population policy is proving to be effective. *China Daily,* October 5, 1989, p. 4.

Gao Shiyu. (1987). Tangdai de Guanji (The government-owned prostitutes). *Shixue Yuekan (Monthly Journal of History)* 1987 (5): 25–30.

Gargan, E. (1988). Newest economics revives the oldest profession. *New York Times,* September 17.

Garside, R. (1981). *Coming alive: China after Mao.* New York: McGraw-Hill.

Ge Hong [A.D. 281–341]. (1965). *Pao Po Tzu (The work of Ko Hung).* Reprinted in Ssu Pu Pei Yao, No. 67. Taipei: Taiwan Chung-hwa Book Co.

Giles, H. A. [1845–1935]. (1967). *A history of Chinese literature* (Supplemented) [With a supplement on the literature of the twentieth century by Liu Wu-chi]. (1st ed., 1901). New York: Frederick Ungar.

Girchner, L.E. (1957). *Erotic aspects of Chinese culture.* Private edition, USA. This work is valuable for the illustrations it contains, many of which would otherwise be extremely difficult to secure.

Gluck, J. (1961). Sex in the art of the Far East. In *The encyclopedia of sexual behavior,* pp. 412–421. (A. Ellis & A. Abarbanel, Eds.) Vol. II. New York: Hawthorne Books.

Gross, A. (1981). Sex through the ages in China. In the walls of China. *SIECUS Report* 10(2 November): 7–8.

Gulik, van, R. H. (1951). *Erotic colour prints of the Ming period, with an essay on Chinese sex life from the Han to the Ch'ing dynasty, B.C. 206–A.D. 1644.* Vol. I, English text; Vol. II, Chinese text; Vol. III, reprint of the Hua-ying-chin-chen album. Private edition of 50 copies, Tokyo, Japan, 1951.

Gulik, van, R. H. (1961). *Sexual life in ancient China: A preliminary survey of Chinese sex and society from ca. 1500 B.C. till A.D. 1644* Leiden: E.J. Brill, 1961; reprint, 1974. Robert H. van Gulik [1910–1967], Litt. D., served as plenipotentiary Minister, became a Master in the Tao, and was the first Westerner to produce an important study of Chinese sexuality. (For the background of this and the above-cited work, see Chapter 1.) This book is a general picture of Chinese sexual life in broad historical and sociological perspectives and attempts to set the record straight concerning foreign misconceptions about sexual life in ancient China. The bibliography itself is an excellent resource, and van Gulik included excerpts from many texts that are difficult to obtain. Many of the sources cited are quite rare and valuable.

Guo, Mo-jo. (1954). *Zhongguo gudai sehui yienjiu (The studies of ancient Chinese society).* Beijing: People's Publishing House.

Hallingby, L. (1981). China: A selected bibliography on sexuality, family planning, and marriage and family. *SIECUS Report* 10(2, November): 9.

Hanan, P. (1981). *The Chinese vernacular story.* Harvard East Asian Series 94. Boston: The President and Fellows of Harvard College.

Harrison, J. A. (1972). *The Chinese empire.* New York: Harcourt Brace Jovanovich.

He Cheng, & Fang Qian. (1989). Yinyang Daocuo de Xingai—zhongguo tongxinglian tanmi. (The sex-love of Yin-Yang inversion: An inquiry into homosexuality in China.) *Qinghai Quncong Yishu* (Bimonthly), No. 103 (April 1989): 2–23.

He Cheng, & Zuo Qi. (1989). Cong Kuangzhou Qianoung Huilai de Maiyinnu. (The prostitutes' forced return from Canton.) *Qinghai Quncong Yishu* (Bimonthly), No. 103 (April, 1989): 24–45, 83.

Hegel, R. E. (1981). *The novel in seventeenth-century China.* New York: Columbia University Press.

Henriques, Fernando. (1962). The prostitution of China. In *Prostitution and society: A survey,* pp. 241–277. New York: Citadel.

Hsia, C. T. (1968). *The classic Chinese novel: A critical introduction.* New York: Columbia University Press.

Hsu, F.L.K. (1953). *Americans and Chinese: Two ways of life.* New York: Henry Schuman.

Hsu Ti-shan [1893–1941]. (1977). *Daojiao Shi (History of Taoism).* 1st ed., 1934; reprint, Taipei, Taiwan: Cowboy Publishing Co, Ltd.

Huai Zhi. (1989). *Luse zi Zheng de Huangse Zui'e (The yellow sins in the green city).* Beijing: Zhongguo Mingjian Wenyi Chubanse.

Huayangzi [a Taoist name]. (Ed.) (1936). *Baoyuandai (The precious waist band)*. (No publishing records.) This is a collection of Taoist books of sexual techniques and regimens, including *She Sheng Pi Phou (Secret Instructions for Regimen)*, edited by Hong Ji; *Fang Shu Hsuan Chi (The Mysterious Essence of Bedchamber Techniques)*, by Chen Xiyi; and *Fang Chung Lien Chi Chieh Yao (Concise Instructions for Strengthening Oneself in the Bedchamber)*, by Hanxuzi [a Taoist name].

Hucker, C.O. (1975). *China's imperial past: An introduction to Chinese history and culture*. Stanford, CA: Stanford University Press.

Humana, C., & Jacobs, J. (1971). *The Ying-Yang: The Chinese way of love*. London: Wingate.

Humana, C., & Wu, W. (1976). "The Ying-Yang: The Chinese way of love." In *Readings in human sexuality: Contemporary perspectives, 1967–77 Edition*, pp. 41–44. (Chad Gordon & Gayle Johnson, Eds.), New York: Harper & Row.

Humana, C., & Wu, W. (1982). *The Chinese way of love*. Hong Kong: CFW Publications. The same book with a different title: *Chinese sex secrets: A look behind the screen*. New York: Gallery Books, 1984.

Hummel, A. W. (Ed.) (1942). *Eminent Chinese in the Ching period (1644–1912)*. 2 Volumes. Washington, DC: U.S. Government Printing Office.

Hyde, J. S. (1982). *Understanding human sexuality*. 2nd ed. New York: McGraw-Hill.

Ishihara, A., & Levy, H. S. (tr.) (1968). *The Tao of sex: An annotated translation of the twenty-eighth section of The essence of medical prescriptions (ISHIMPO)*. New York: Harper & Row. See Levy & Ishihara, 1989.

Jiang, X. Y. (1988). *"Xin" zhai gudai zhongguo ("Sex" in ancient China)*. Xi'an: Shianxi Scientific and Technical Publishing House.

Jiang, Y. F., et al. (1988). Sex education in Shanghai. *Shanghai Pictorial* (Bimonthly), No. 2: 12–15.

Kang Suzhen. (1988a). *Wo de Jinu Shenghuo (My prostitute's life)*. Shijiazhuang: Hobei People's Publishing House. It was said by the publisher that this book is the first autobiography of a prostitute in Chinese history. However, her story was published at the same time, under another title, in the style of a classical Chinese novel (see next citation).

Kang Suzhen. (1988b). *Qinglouhen (Green house hatred)*. Harbin: Helongjiang People's Publishing House.

Kargren, B. (Trans.) (1950). *The book of odes*. Stockholm: Museum of Far Eastern Antiquities.

Kel, A., & Ruan, F. F. (1987). A complete list of sexual activities. In *The sex master*. Unpublished manuscript.

Kristof, N. D. (1990). "Curing" homosexuals in China. *San Francisco Chronicle*, January 31, 1990.

Kronhausen, P., & Kronhausen, E. (Eds.) (1968). *Erotic art: A survey of erotic fact and fancy in the fine arts*. 41 color plates & 400 black and white plates. China, pp. 240–259. New York: Bell Publishing Co,.

Kronhausen, P. & Kronhausen, E. (1978). *The complete book of erotic art*. China. Vol. I, pp. 240–259; Vol. II, pp. 189–218. New York: Bell Publishing Co.

Kuhn, F. (1965). *The before midnight scholar (Jou Pu Tuan of Li Yu)*. London: Deutsch.

Latourette, K. S. (1972). *The Chinese: Their history and culture*. 4th ed., New York: Macmillan.

Legge, James. (Trans., 1899) (1963). *The I-Ching: The book of changes*. Reprint, New York: Dover.

Legge, James. (Trans., 1871) (1971). *The she king (The book of poetry)*. Reprint, Taipei, Taiwan: Wen Shi Zhe Press.

Legge, James. (Trans., 1892) (1971). *Confucian analects: The great learning and the doctrine of the mean*. Reprint, New York: Dover.

Legge, James. (Trans., 1892) (1983). *The four books*. Reprint, Taipei, Taiwan: Culture Book Co.

Levy, H. S. (1965). *Chinese footbinding: The history of a curious erotic custom*. New York: Bell Publishing Co. An extensively illustrated history of footbinding, with emphasis on the esoteric and erotic aspects. It is a thorough treatment of a unique Chinese custom which has long aroused curiosity in the West.

Levy, H. S. (Trans.) (1967). *The gay quarters at Nanking (Diverse records of Wooden Bridge)* Privately printed, Yokohoma.

Levy, H. S. (Ed. & Trans.) (1974). *Chinese sex jokes in traditional times.* Taipei: The Orient Cultural Service.

Levy, H. S., & Ishihara, A. (Trans.) (1989). *The Tao of sex: The essence of medical prescriptions (Ishimpo).* Illustrator: R. Stodart. 3rd rev. ed. Lower Lake, CA: Integral Publishing. See Ishihara & Levy (1968).

Li, Jingwei; Cheng, Zhifan; & Ruan, Fangfu. (Eds.) (1987). *Chinese encyclopedia of medicine: Medical history.* Shanghai: Shanghai Scientific and Technological Publishing House.

Li Shihua, & Shen Denhui. (Eds.) (1987). *Daozang Yangshenshu Shizhong (Ten books on the way to preserve one's health, from the Taoist Canon).* Beijing: Zhongyi Guji Chubanshe. *Daozang* (the *Taoist Canon*) is a vast collection of Taoist scriptures, which consists of 5,485 volumes comprising some 200,000 pages, and is divided into more than 1,600 books.

Lieh-Mak, F., O'Hoy, K. M., & Luk, S. L. (1983). Lesbianism in the Chinese of Hong Kong. *Archives of Sexual Behavior* 12(1): 21–30.

Lin, Yutang. (1935). *My country and my people.* New York: John Day/Reynal & Hitchcock.

Ling Meng-chu [A.D. 1580–1644]. (1982a). *P'o-an ching-ch'i (Pa-An Ching-Chi) (Striking the table in amazement at the wonders)* Reprint, Shanghai: Shanghai Gu-Ji Publisher.

Ling Meng-chu. (1982b). *Erh-k'o P'o-an ching-ch'i (Erh-Kuo Pa-an Ching-chi) (The second collection of striking the table in amazement at the wonders).* Reprint, Shanghai: Shanghai Gu-Ji Publisher.

Liu Cunren. (1982). *Lendun suo jian Zhongguo xiaoshuo Shumu tiyao (A descriptive bibliography of Chinese works of fiction seen in London)* Beijing: Bibliographic and Literature Publishing House.

Liu Da-lin. (1987). Science of sex and liberation of women. *The Frontier of Social Sciences* (1): 120–125.

Liu Hsu. (Ed.) (1975). *Chiu Tang Shu (Old history of the Tang dynasty, A.D. 618–906).* Reprint, Beijing: Zhonghua Books.

Liu, I. C. (1976). *Shih-shuo hsin-yu (A new account of tales of the world).* (Trans. R.B. Mather) Minneapolis: University of Minnesota Press. (Original work published during the fifth century A.D.)

Liu, Z. (1984). *Two years in the melting pot.* San Francisco: China Books & Periodicals.

Liu, Zhong-yi. (1987). Difference in concept of sex between the East and West. Unpublished paper.

Lu Dongbin [A.D. ?–789]. (1598). *Chi-Chi-Chen-Ching (True manual of the "perfected equalization").* (The complete title is *Chun-yang yen-cheng fou-yu-ti-chun chi-chi-chen-ching [True classic of the complete union, by the all-assisting Lord Chun-yang]*) This work is attributed to Lu Dongbin, also called Lu Chun-yang (Pure Yang), Taoist immortal. He is said to have lived during the Sung dynasty and later was made one of the Pa-hsian, the well-known set of the Taoist Eight Immortals. It is annotated by Deng Xixian (Tzu Chin Kuang Yao Ta Hsien, the Great Immortal of the Purple-Gold Splendor), a famous Ming dynasty Taoist monk. This is a handbook of Taoists' sexual techniques (physiological alchemy). It was partially translated into English by van Gulik in his *Sexual Life in Ancient China* (cited above). The Chinese text used here was hand-copied from a Ming dynasty blockprint [A.D. 1598] in the Beijing Library Rare Books Division by Fang Fu Ruan, in 1985. The text may also be found in Tan Ching, (Ed.) (1986): *Zhongguo gu-yan xi-ping cong-kan (Chinese Classical Erotic Rare Book Series),* No. 30.

Lu Dongbin. (Before 1850). *Lu Tsu Wu Phien (The Taoist Patriarch Lu Dongbin's five poetical essays on sexual techniques)*. Attrib. Lu Dongbin. Annotated by Fu Chin-chhuan, reprinted in *Cheng Tao Pi Shu Shihchi Chung (Seventeen Types of Secret Books on the Verification of the Tao)*, ed. by Fu Chin-chhuan in the early nineteenth century. A booklet in which Taoist sexual techniques are described in poems.

Lu Guangrong, Lou Yugang, & Wu Jiachun. (Eds.) (1987). Daozang *Qigongshu Shizhong (Ten Books on Chi-Kung from the Taoist Canon)*. Beijing: Zhongyi Guji Chubanshe. See Li & Shen (1987).

Lu, H. C. (Trans.) (1978). *A complete translation of the yellow emperor's classic of internal medicine and the difficult classic*, Vancouver, Canada: The Academy of Oriental Heritage.

Lu, H. C. (1986): *Chinese system of food cures: Prevention and remedies*. New York: Sterling.

Lu Hsun [pen name of Chou Shu-jen, 1881–1936]. (Trans. G. Yang & H.Y. Yang) (1976). *A brief history of Chinese fiction*. 3rd ed. Beijing: Foreign Languages Press.

Ma Yau-Woon, & Lau, J.S.M. (1978). *Traditional Chinese stories*. New York: Columbia University Press.

Martin, R. (Trans.) (1966). *Jou Pu Tuan (The prayer mat of flesh)*. New York: Grove Press. One of the best classical Chinese erotic novels. Originally published by an anonymous using the pseudonym of "Mr. Qingyin," it is attributed to Li Yu [A.D. 1611–1679], a famous dramatist, novelist, and essayist. First published in 1634. This English edition was translated from the German version by author Dr. Franz Kuhn [1884–1961] and published by Verlage Die Waage, Zurich, in 1959. It contains 60 illustrations.

Meisner, M. (1986). *Mao's China and after: A history of the People's Republic* (A revised and expanded edition of *Mao's China*). New York: Free Press.

Mitchell, S. (Trans.) (1988). *Tao Te Ching* (A New English Version, with Foreword and Notes). New York: Harper & Row.

Money, J. (1977). Chapter 39: Peking: The Sexual Revolution. In *Handbook of Sexology* (J. Money & H. Musaph, Eds.), pp. 643–550. Amsterdam: Excerpta Medica.

Murstein, B. I. (1974). *Love, sex, and marriage through the ages*. Chapter 20: Marriage in China: Past and present, pp. 467–485. New York: Springer.

Needham, J. (1956). *Science and civilisation in China*. Vol. 2, Sect. 8–18. Cambridge, UK: Cambridge University Press.

Needham, J. (1983). *Science and civilisation in China*. Vol. 5, Part V: Spagyrical discovery and invention: Physiological alchemy. Sexuality and the role of theories of generation. Cambridge, UK: Cambridge University Press.

Norrgard, L. (1990). Opening the Hong Kong closet. *Out/Look* (National Lesbian and Gay Quarterly) 2(3, Winter):56–61.

Ouyang Hsiu [A.D. 1007–1072] and Sung Chhi [A.D. 998–1061]. (Eds.) (1975). *Hsin Tang Shu (New history of the Tang dynasty, A.D. 618–906)*. Reprint, Beijing: Zhonghua Books.

Pan, G. D. (1947). Translator's Notes and Appendix. In H. Ellis, *Psychology of sex* (Chinese translation edition, trans. G. D. Pan), pp. 249–255, 380–406. Shanghai: Commercial Press.

Parker, W. (1971). *Homosexuality: A selective bibliography of 3,000 items*. Metuchen, NJ: Scarecrow Press.

Parker, W. (1977). *Homosexuality bibliography: Supplement, 1970–1975*. Metuchen, NJ: Scarecrow Press.

Parker, W. (1985). *Homosexuality bibliography: Second supplement, 1976–1982*. Metuchen, NJ: Scarecrow Press.

Pelton, L. C. (1982). A family physician views sexual medicine in the People's Republic. *Sexual Medicine Today* January, pp. 23–24.

Pouly, I. B., & Edgerton, M. T. (1986). The gender identity movement: A growing surgical-psychiatric liaison. *Archives of Sexual Behavior* 15: 315–329.

Qian, Xuian-tung. (1982). Reply to Mr. Gu, Jie-kang. In *Gushipian (The critical analysis of the history of ancient China)*. Vol. I. Shanghai: Shanghai Guji Publishing House.

Rawsan, P. (1968). *Erotic art of the East*. New York: Prometheus.

Rawsan, P. (1981). *Oriental erotic art*. Chapter 3: China. pp. 75–124. New York: A & W Publications.

Reischauer, E. O., & Fairbank, J. K. (1960). *East Asia: The great tradition*. Boston: Houghton Mifflin.

Ronan, A. C., & Needham, J. (1978): *The shorter science and civilisation in China: An abridgement of Joseph Needham's original text*. Vol. 1 (Vols. I and II of the major series). Cambridge, UK: Cambridge University Press.

Ruan, Fang Fu [using pseud. C. Z. Yang]. (1976a). One of the most brilliant achievements in the preparation and use of sex hormones in eleventh century China. *Dongwu Xuiebao (Acta Zoologica Sinica)*, 22: 192–196.

Ruan, Fang Fu [using pseud. C. Z. Yang]. (1976b). Shen Kuo (A.D. 1031–1095) and medicine. *Beijing Yixueyuan Xuiebao (Journal of Peking Medical College)* (3):189–193.

Ruan, Fang Fu. (1977). Medicine and health in the primitive society. *Beijing Yixueyuan Xuiebao (Journal of Peking Medical College)* (3):189–191, and 196).

Ruan, Fang Fu. (1979; 1983). *Xingjisu de faxian (Discovery of the sex hormones)*. 1st ed., 1979; expanded 2nd ed., 1983. Beijing: Science Press.

Ruan, Fang Fu. (1984). *Yixue xinlun (New treatise on medicine)*. Harbin: Heilongjiang Scientific and Technological Publishing House.

Ruan, Fang Fu [using pseud. J. M. Hua] (1985a). Homosexuality: An unsolved puzzle. *Zhu Nin Jiankang (To Your Good Health)*, 1985(3), 14–15.

Ruan, Fang Fu. (Ed.) (1985b). *Xing zhishi shouce (Handbook of sex knowledge)*. Beijing: Scientific and Technological Literature Publishing House. This book consists of 18 chapters. Chapter titles are as follows: (1) Science of Sex; (2) Sex Organs; (3) Sex Hormones; (4) Sexual Development; (5) Psychology of Sex; (6) Sexual Response; (7) Sexual Behaviors; (8) Sexual Hygiene; (9) Sexual Dysfunctions; (10) Sexual Varieties; (11) Sex Crime; (12) Sex and Marriage; (13) Sex and Reproduction; (14) Sex in Illness; (15) Sex and Drugs; (16) Sex in the Aged; (17) Sex Therapy; and (18) Sex Education. Wu Jie-ping and twenty other eminent professors were invited as advisors and gynecology professor Zhang Li-zu and twenty other professionals were invited as contributors. The volume was the first and the only comprehensive sex handbook published in mainland China since 1949.

Ruan, F. F., & Bullough, V. L. (1988). The First case of transsexual surgery in Mainland China. *The Journal of Sex Research* 25: 546–547.

Ruan, F. F., & Bullough, V. L. (1989a). Sex in China. *Medical Aspects of Human Sexuality* 23: 59–62.

Ruan, F. F., & Bullough, V. L. (1989b). Sex repression in contemporary China. In *Building a world community: Humanism in the 21st century*, pp. 198–201. (P. Kurtz, Ed.), Buffalo, NY: Prometheus Books.

Ruan, F. F., & Chong, K.R. (1987). Gay life in China. *The Advocate* 470 (April 14), 28–31.

Ruan, F. F., & Tsai, Y. M. (1987). Male homosexuality in the traditional Chinese literature. *Journal of Homosexuality* 14: 21–33.

Ruan, F. F., & Tsai, Y. M. (1988). Male homosexuality in contemporary Mainland China. *Archives of Sexual Behavior* 17: 189–199.

Ruan, F. F., Bullough, V. L., & Tsai, Y. M. (1989). Male transsexualism in mainland China. *Archives of Sexual Behavior* 18: 517–522.

Samshasha [or Xiao Mingxiong, pseudonyms]. (1984). *Zhong guo tongxing'ai shilu (History of homosexuality in China)*, Hong Kong: Pink Triangle Press.

Samshasha. (1989). *Tungxing'ai wenti sanshijiang (Thirty questions about homosexuality)*. Hong Kong: Yiuwo.

Sankar, A. (1986). Sisters and brothers, lovers and enemies: Marriage resistance in South Kwangtung. *Anthropology and Homosexual Behavior* 69–81.

Scott, J. (Ed. & Trans.) (1972). *Love and protest: Chinese poems from the sixth century B.C. to the seventeenth century A.D.* New York: Harper & Row.

Siqiao Qushi. [anon., pseud., 17th century]. (1987). *Ge Lian Hua Ying (The flower's shadow behind the curtain).* Originally published ca. 1691 A.D., a Ching dynasty blockprinted edition from Hunan Province, reprinted 1987, 2 volumes. Taipei, Taiwan: Tan-Ch'ing Book Company.

Shui Shui. (1989). Nu Tongxinglian Gongsi. (Lesbians' Company.) In *Junlu Yanqing (The love story in the military tour)*, pp. 66–95. Shengyang: Liaoning Mingzu Press.

Shulman, A. G. (1979). Absence of venereal disease in the People's Republic of China. *The Western Journal of Medicine* 130: 469–471.

Sierles, F. (1982). *Clinical behavioral science.* Jamaica, NY: Spectrum.

de Smedt, M. (Trans. P. Lane) (1981). *Chinese eroticism.* New York: Crescent Books.

Smith, B. (1974). *Erotic art of the masters: The 18th, 19th & 20th centuries.* "China," pp. 22–27, 84–93. Secaucus, NJ: Lyle Stuart.

Sun Kaiti. (1958). *Riben Dongjing suo jian Zhongguo xiaoshuo Shumu [tiyao] (A [descriptive] bibliography of Chinese works of fiction seen in Tokyo).* First ed.: Peiping: Peiping National Library, 1932. The newer edition deletes the word "tiyao (descriptive)" from the title. Shanghai: Shang-tsa chupansche, 1953. Beijing: People's Literature Publishing House.

Sun Kaiti. (1982). *Zhongguo tongsu xiaoshuo shumu (A catalogue of Chinese works of popular fiction).* First ed.: Peiping: National Peiping Library, 1932; revised ed.: Beijing: Tso-chia chu-pan-she, 1958; new ed., Beijing: People's Literature Publishing House.

Sun Simiao [A.D. 581–682]. (1982). *Bei Ji Qian Jin Yao Fang (Prescriptions worth a thousand pieces of gold for emergencies).* Reprint, Beijing: People's Medical Publishing House.

Ssuma Chhien. [146–86 BC]. (1959). *Shi Ji (Historical Records)* (from early time to 99 B.C., first ed., 90 B.C.). 130 vols. Reprint, Beijing: Zhonghua Books Co.

Stafford, P. (1967). *Sexual behavior in the Communist World.* "China," pp. 13–57. New York: Julian Press.

Strong, B., & DeVault, C. (1988). *Understanding our sexuality.* 2nd ed. St. Paul, MN: West.

Tan Chengpi. (1984). *Guban xijian xiaoshuo huikao (Bibliographical studies of Rare Fictions in Old Editions.)* Hongzhou: Zhejiang Literaturrre and Art Publishing House.

Tan Ching. (Ed.) (1986). *Zhong-guo gu-yan xi-ping cong-kan (Chinese Classical Erotic Rare Book Series).* 44 titles [No. 1–44] in 22 volumes. Taipei, Taiwan: Tan-ch'ing Book Company.

Tan Ching. (Ed.) (1986–#19). *Zhu-lin ye-shi (Unofficial History of the Bamboo Garden).* By an anonymous Ching dynasty author, 6 rolls, 16 chapters. Reprint, Taipei, Taiwan: Tan-ch'ing Books Company.

Tan Ching. (Ed.) (1986–#21). *Rou Pu Tuan (Jou Pu Tuan, The prayer mat of flesh).* By Qingyin (anon., pseud., Ming dynasty) Reprint, Taipei, Taiwan: Tan-ch'ing Book Company. See R. Martin (1967).

Tannahill, R. (1980). *Sex in history.* Chapter 7: China, pp. 164–198. New York: Stein & Day.

Teng Hsi-Hsien. (1598). *Hsiu Chen Yen I (A popular exposition of the methods of regenerating the primary vitalities).* The complete title is *Tzu-chin-Kuang-yueh-ta-hsien-hsiu-chen-yeni (Explanation of the meaning of the cultivation of truth, by the great immortal of the purple-gold splendor).* By Teng Hsi-hsien (Tzu Chin Kuang Yao Ta Hsien, the great immortal of the purple-gold splendor), a famous Ming dynasty Taoist monk. A handbook of Taoist sexual techniques (physiological alchemy), it was partially translated into English by van Gulik in *Sexual Life in Ancient China* (cited ab). The Chinese text used here was hand-copied from a Ming dynasty blockprint (A.D. 1598) in the Beijing Library Rare Books Division by Fang Fu Ruan, in 1985.

Tien, Yi. (Ed.) (1985). *Ming-Qing Shan-ban shiao-shuo cong-kan: yan-qing shiao-shuo zuan-ji (Ming-Ching Rare Fictions Series: Erotic Novels Series)*. 25 titles [No. 212–236] in 37 books. Taipei, Taiwan: T'ien-yi Ch'u-pan-she.

Tsao, Hsueh Chin [1715?–1763]. (1982). *Honglou Meng (Dream of the Red Chamber)*. Reprint, (A.D. 1st ed., 1791), 3 vols. Beijing: People's Literature Press.

Tuveson, R. (1982). First gay tour of China. *Mandate*, December: 10–13, 62–63.

Veith, I. (Trans.) (1972). *The yellow emperor's classic of internal medicine*. (paper ed.). Berkeley, CA: University of California Press.

Waley, A. (Trans.) (1937). *The book of songs*. London: Allen & Unwin.

Waley, A. (Trans.) (1958). *The way and its power: A study of the Tao Te Ching and its place in Chinese thought*. New York: Grove Press.

Wan Ruixiong. (1988). Xingai Da Bianzou—Guanyu Zhongguo de Tongxinglian Wenti ("The bigger variations of sex and love—About the problems of homosexuality in China."), pp. 78–109. In *Nu Shi Ren Tan (The ten women's tales)*, Wen Bo, Ed., Beijing: China Social Sciences Press.

Wang Liqi [Hsiao-ch'uan]. (Ed.) (1981). *Yuan Ming Ch'ing san-tai chin-hui hsiao-shuo hsi-chu shih-iiao (Historical Materials of the banned fictions and plays in the Yuan, Ming, and Ching Dynasties)*. Enlarged ed. Shanghai: Shanghai Guji Chubanshe.

Wang Ming. (Ed.) (1960). *Taipingjing Hejiao (Combined proofreading and correction of the Canon of Peace and Tranquility)*. Beijing: Zhonghua Books.

Wang Ming. (1982). The new explanation of the "Hsien kua" in *I-Ching*. In *Zhongguo Zhexue (Chinese philosophy)*, Vol. 7. Beijing: Sanlian Books.

Wang Minghui. (1989). *Zhongyi Xingyixue (Traditional Chinese sexual medicine)*. Wuhan: Hubei Science and Technique Publishing House.

Wang Shunu. (1934). *Zhongguo Changji Shi (A history of prostitutes in China)*. Shanghai: Shenghuo Books Co.

Wang Wen-bin, Zhao Zhi-yi, & Tan Ming-xin. (1957). *Xing-di-zhi-shi (Knowledge of Sex)*. Beijing: Popular Science Publishing House.

Wang Hongyan & Zhou Jiren. (Eds.) (1983). *Wudaisong Xiaoshuoxian (Selected short stories of the Five Dynasties and Song dynasty [A.D. 907–1279]*. Zhengzhou: Zhongzhou Publishing House.

Ware, J.R. (Trans. & Ed.) (1966). *Alchemy, medicine, religion in the China of A.D. 320: The Nei P'ian of Ko Hung (Pao-p'u tzu)*. Republication, 1981. Cambridge, MA: M.I.T. Press.

Watson, B. (Trans.) (1964). *Han Fei Tzu: Basic writing*. New York: Columbia University Press. (Original work published third century B.C.)

Wei Cheng (Ed.). (1973). *Sui Shu (History of the Sui dynasty)*. Reprint, Beijing: Zhonghua Books.

Wei, Y., & Wong, A. (1949). A study of 500 prostitutes in Shanghai. *International Journal of Sexology* 2: 234–238.

Weixing Shiguan Zhaizhu [pseudonym meaning the master of the study of sexual conception of history.] (1964). *Lishi Xing Wenxian (Historical literature of sex)*. 2 volumes. Hong Kong: Yuzhou (Universe) Publishing House.

Weixing Shiguan Zhaizhu. (1967). *Zhongguo Tongxinglian mishi (Secret history of homosexuality in China)*. 2nd ed. (1st ed., 1964), 2 volumes. Hong Kong: Yuzhou (Universe) Publishing House.

Weinberg, M. S., & Bell, A. P. (1972). *Homosexuality: An annotated bibliography*. New York: Harper & Row.

Weisskopf, M. (1980). China's latest "Red Book" is all about sex. *Washington Post*, November 12.

Wen Bo. (Ed.) (1988a). *Nu Shi Ren Tan (The ten women's tales)*. Beijing: China Social Sciences Press.

Wen Bo. (Ed.) (1988b). *Zhongguoren de Hunyin (Marriage among the Chinese people)*. Beijing: China Social Sciences Press.

Wenhua. (Ed.) (1984). *Zhongguo Mingjian Tongsu Xiaoshuo (Chinese Classic Folk Popular Novelettes)*. Taipei: Wenhua Tushu Co.

Wolf, A. P. (1966). Childhood association, sexual attraction and the incest taboo: A Chinese case. *American Anthropoligist*, New (2nd) Series 68:4 (August): 883–898.

Wu, C. Z. (1988). *The studies of crimes related to sex, love, and marriage*. Beijing: Beijing Office of Guiding Group of Philosophy and Social Sciences Programs.

Wu Jie-ping. (1980). Let young people learn physiological and hygiene knowledge. *Jiankang-bao (Health Newspaper)*, May 4.

Wu Jie-ping. (1987). Speech at a national meeting, reported in *People's Daily* (Overseas Edition) March 5, 1987.

Wu, L. T. (1961). Sexual life in the Orient, pp. 794–801. In *The Encyclopedia of Sexual Behavior* (A. Ellis & A. Abarbanel, Eds.). Volume II. New York: Hawthorn Books.

Wu, Z. G., Huang, Z. L., & Mei, S. W. (1981). *Peking opera and Mei Lanfang: A guide to China's traditional theatre and the art of its great master*. Beijing: New World Press.

Wuxia Ameng [anon., pseud., 17th century]. (Ed.) (1909). *Duan Xiu Pian (Tuan-hsiu-pien, Records of the Cut Sleeve)*. Reprinted in *Xiang yan Cong Shu (Hsiang-yen-ts'ung-shu, Collected Writings on Fragrant Elegance)*, Section 9, Volume 2. Shanghai: China Books Co. This book summarizes literary data on male homosexuality by describing fifty well-known cases from Chinese official histories and unofficial histories.

Xia Zhengnong. (Ed.) (1980). *Cihai (The sea of words)*. Shanghai: Cishu Cubanshe.

Xiao Xiaoshen [anon., pseud., Ming dynasty]. (1957). *Jin Ping Mei Cihua (Chin P'ing Mei Tz'u-hua, The golden lotus, or Chin P'ing Mei: The adventurous history of Hsi Man and his six wives)*. One hundred chapters, in 21 vols. Beijing: Wenxue Guji Kanxingshe. One of the four greatest Chinese novels. The first edition may have been published in A.D. 1610. This 1957 reprint is based on the 1617 version, which contains the greatest amount of explicit erotic description.

Xin Yue Zhu Ren [pseudonym]. (1810?). *Yi-chun Xiang-zhi (Pleasant spring and fragrant character)*. The edition used for this book is a handwritten copy stored in the Beijing Library.

Yang, H.X. (1988). *Xing Xinli (Psychology of sex)*. Shijiazhuang: Hebei People's Publishing House.

Yang, R.F.S., & Levy, H.S. (Trans.). (1971). *Monks and nuns in a sea of sins*. Sino-Japanese sexology classics series, Vol. II. Washington, DC: The Warm-Soft Village Press.

Yao, L. X. (Ed.) (1940). *P'ing-wai chih-yen (Papers and reference materials on Chin P'ing Mei)*. Tianjin: Tianjin Books. Yao Lin Xi (Ling-hsi) is a famous researcher of Chinese sexology, especially the custom of footbinding. This book contains a valuable glossary by the editor.

Yao, L. X. (1941). *Siwuxie Shaoji* (or *Yan Hai, The sea of words*), Tianjin: Tianjin Books. This book is a comprehensive annotated collection of Chinese erotic fiction, stories, poems, historical records, essays, and other materials.

Yasuyori, T. (Ed.) (1955). *Yi Xin Fang (I-hsin-fang)*. In Japanese: *I-shim-po (The essence of medical prescriptions)* Vol. 28: Fang Nei (Within the bedroom), Reprint, Beijing: People's Medical Publishing House, 1955, pp. 633–659. See text for a complete description of this work. Since most of the excerpts it contains are preserved nowhere else, this text is of incalculable value. *Tao of sex* by Ishihara, A. & Levy, H. S., 1968 (cited) is an English translation. *I-shim-po* is also the major source of Volume 1 of Yeh's *Shuang Mei Ching An Tshung Shu (Double plum-tree collection)* (see the following).

Ye Gong-shao. (1983). Premier Zhou was concerned with sex education. *Fu-mu Bi-du (Required readings for parents)*, No. 4, 1983.

Yeh Te-hui. (Ed.) (1914). *Shuang Mei Ching An Tshung Shu (Double plum-tree collection)*. Vol. 1, Changsha: Guan-gu-tung. See text for a discussion of the history and contents of this important collection.

Yi Jiancun. (1980). Annotated notes on talks on the super Tao in the world: Seven hurts and eight advantages. *Hunan Zhongyi Xueyuan Xuebao (Journal of Human Traditional Chinese Medical College)*. 1980(1): 27–32.

Yi Ni. (1988). *Yangguang Xia de Shikuao (Pondering under a shining sun)*. Beijing: Zhongguo Wenlian Chuban gongshi.

Yu Guangyuan. (Ed.) (1956). Xing-zhi-shi (Sex knowledge). Shanghai: Shanghai Health Publishing House.

Zhang Beiduan [Ziyang Zhenren, Chang Po-tuan, A.D. 984–1082]. (1987). *Wu Chen Phien (Poetical essay on realising the necessity of regenerating the primary vitalities)*. Composed in about A.D. 1075. Reprinted in Lu, Lou, & Wu (eds., 1987): *Daozang Qigongshu Shizhong (Ten books on Chi-Kung from the Taoist Canon)*, pp. 60–78.

Zhang Junying. (1641). *Ren Jing Jing (The classic of the human mirror)*. Xuzhou: Jingshitang.

Zhang, M. C. (1950). *Materialist sexology*. Shanghai: Time Books.

Zhang Mingcheng [1934–]. (1974). *A history of traditional Chinese medicine: Herbs, acupuncture, and regimen*. In Japanese. Tokyo: Hisaho Books.

Zhang Sanfeng. (Before 1850). *San Feng Tan Chueh (Zhang sanfeng's instructions in the physiological alchemy, The healing techniques of Master Chang San-Feng)*. Reprinted in Cheng Tao Pi Shu Shihchi Chung (Seventeen types of secret books on the verification of the Tao), Fu Chin-chhuan, Ed. Early 19th century. A handbook of Taoist sexual techniques (physiological alchemy) by Zhang Sanfeng, a famous Taoist monk of the Liu-Sung (?) dynasty.

Zhao Liangpi [Ziyang Daoren]. (Before 1850). *Hsuan Wei Hshin In (Mental images of the mysteries and subtleties of sexual techniques, or The sacred seal in the heart)*, Volume I & II. Reprinted in *Cheng Tao Pi Shu Shihchi Chung (Seventeen types of secret books on the verification of the Tao)*, Fu Chin-chhuan, Ed. Early 19th century. Another handbook of Taoist sexual techniques. Zhao was a Ming dynasty Taoist.

Zhonghua Tushu Jicheng Bianjisuo [Chinese Book Collection Institute] (Eds.) (1925). *Shanghai funu niejingtai (The mirror of sins of women in Shanghai)*. 4 vols., 7th ed. (1st ed., 1918). Shanghai: Zhonghua Tushu Jicheng Company.

Zhou, Shaoxian [1908–]. (1982). *Daojia yu Shenxian (Taoists and immortals)*. 3rd ed. Taipei, Taiwan: Chung Hwa Book Company, Ltd.

Zhou Yimiu. (1989). *Zhongguo gudai fangshi yangshengxie (The studies of sexual life and regimen)*. Shenyang: Zhongwei Wenhua Publishing Co. Appended to this book were the entire texts, with modern Chinese translations, of three earliest Chinese sex booklets: *Shi-wan (Ten questions and answers)*, *He-yin-yang-fang (Methods of intercourse between Yin and Yang)*, and *Tian-xia-zhi-tao-tan (Lectures on the super Tao in the universe)*.

Zhu Xing. (1980). *Jin Ping Mei Kaozheng (A textual research on the golden lotus)*. Tianjin: Beihua Wenyi Chubanshe.

Zhu Zhijia [pen name of Jin Xiongbai, 1903–]. (1971). *Cungjiang huayuehen (A memoir of sexual life in Shanghai)*. Hong Kong: Wu Xinji Press.

Zmiewski, P. (Ed.) (1985). *Fundamentals of Chinese medicine* Brookline, MA: Paradigm Publications.

*   *   *   *   *

Chinese language newspapers published in the United States, Mainland China, Taiwan, or Hong Kong, and cited in this book:

Central Daily News (Zhongyany Ribao) International Edition, published in Taipei, Taiwan.

Centre Daily News (Zhong Bao) published in Long Island, NY; Los Angeles, CA; San Francisco, CA; Houston, TX; and Canada; mainly circulated in United States and Canada.

Da Gong Daily News (Da Gong Bao), a newspaper published in Hong Kong but controlled by the Chinese Communist Party and the government of the People's Republic of China.

Health Newspaper (Jian-kang-bao), a public health and medical newspaper published in Beijing by the central government.

International Daily News (Guoji Bibao) published in Los Angeles, CA, and San Francisco, CA; mainly circulated in the United States.

People's Daily (Renming Ribao) Published in Beijing by the central government of the PRC, controlled by the Chinese Communist Party, circulated in China.

People's Daily—Overseas Edition (Renming Ribao—Haiwaiban), the foreign edition of the newspaper cited above; also circulates in China.

Sing Pao Daily News (Cheng Bao) [American Edition], a Hong Kong newspaper printed and circulated in San Francisco, CA, and other cities in the United States and Canada.

Sing Tao Daily (Xing Dao Ribao), a daily newspaper transmitted via satellite from Hong Kong, printed and circulated in San Francisco, CA, and other cities.

Sing Tao Evening News (Xing Dao Wanbao), published in Hong Kong.

World Journal (Shijie Ribao), published in New York, NY; Los Angeles, CA; San Francisco, CA; Houston, TX; and Canada; mainly circulated in the United States and Canada.

The Young China Daily (Shaonian Zhongguo Chengbao), published in San Francisco, controlled by the Chinese Kuomingtang.

*   *   *   *   *

English language newspapers and magazines published in Mainland China, Taiwan, or Hong Kong, and cited in this book:

China Daily, owned by the Chinese central government, published in Beijing, controlled by the CCP, circulated both in China and abroad.

Sing Tao International (English Supplement of *Sing Tao Daily,* cited above).

Index